Beyond Diagnosis

Perspective in Medicine and the
Human Experience

Dr. Francisco M. Torres, MD

Copyright © 2024 by Dr. Francisco Torres, MD

All rights reserved.

No portion of this book may be reproduced in any form without written permission from the publisher or author, except as permitted by U.S. copyright law.

ISBN: 979-8-9905418-0-1

Contents

Foreword	VI
Introduction	X
1. The Early Days of Telemedicine	1
2. Telemedicine Does Not Absolve Us as Doctors	2
3. When Textbooks Are Not Enough	6
4. Why We Should Pay More Attention To Our Intuition	8
5. When the Doctor Understands More Than You Know	11
6. The Importance of Non-Judgmental Empathy	13
7. Toeing the Line as a Healthcare Provider	17
8. Are We Too Scared to Talk to Our Patients About Their Weight?	19
9. When Nutrition and Psychology Collide	23
10. We Cannot Ignore Nutrition's Impact on Both Pain and Obesity	25
11. Are We Listening?	30

12.	Not Listening Carefully to a Vulnerable Patient Can Become a Matter of Life or Death	32
13.	The Power of Distance Healing	35
14.	How Technology is Transforming Medicine and Making Distance Healing a Reality	36
15.	If We Want Change, We Must Pay Attention to Opportunities	40
16.	Why Taking Risks is Worth it: a Doctor's Journey from Uncertainty to Opportunity	42
17.	Blazing Your Own Career Path	46
18.	Combining Academic Medicine and Private Practice: a Success Story	47
19.	When Death Comes for the Doctor	51
20.	Why This Doctor Imagines His Own Funeral Every Year	53
21.	When It Actually Is a Zebra	57
22.	Finding Hope and Relief: a Physical Therapist's Journey with Chronic Pain and Ehlers-Danlos Syndrome (EDS)	59
23.	When Surgery Isn't Necessary	63
24.	Optimize Your Knee Injury Recovery Without Surgery	65
25.	When Respect Becomes a Challenge	70
26.	Patient Respect in Medicine: Ensuring Well-Being and Trust	71
27.	Creating a Legacy: Selfish or Selfless?	76
28.	What Does it Mean to Have a Legacy As a Doctor?	78

29.	What Kids Can Teach Doctors	82
30.	What My Children Have Taught Me About Medicine	83
31.	Are We Rational In Our Use of Psychiatric Assessments?	87
32.	Debating the Role of Psychiatric Assessments in Medical Decisions	88
33.	Is Ozempic All It's Cracked Up to Be?	93
34.	Ozempic: Miracle Drug or a Band-Aid for Obesity?	94
35.	We Are Never Too Old to Learn New Tricks	98
36.	Lessons From Treating a Transgender Patient	100
37.	Is There a Class on How to Give Bad News?	104
38.	A Intern's Journey in Delivering Tough Diagnoses	105
39.	When Doctors are Unprepared	109
40.	From Pain Management to Port au Prince: a Doctor's Journey in Disaster Relief	110
41.	The Human Element	114
42.	Unlocking Compassion: Lessons from a Prison Clinic	115
43.	Conclusion	119
44.	About the Author	122
45.	You Might Also Enjoy These Books by Dr. Torres...	123
46.	Provocative Thoughts for Daily Living	124

Foreword

By Dr. Felix Linetsky

I began my medical practice over 45 years ago in Ukraine, which was part of the Soviet Union at the time. In those days, doctors were often paid the same salaries as factory workers or even less. We practiced medicine out of a passion for healing. It was less scientific than in the USA, but it was also a humanistic art form.

Dr. Torres' book delves deeply into these human aspects of medicine. Most of his essays focus on the relationship between doctors and their patients. That relationship is at the core of our profession: one person healing another. Statistics and empirical research have unquestionably modernized, advanced, and improved this field. Still, Dr. Torres' book reminds us that medical inquiry cannot stop at a collection of interchangeable laboratory values.

Decades of rigorous research have taught us that human traits and experiences can significantly impact care outcomes. This has resulted in a push for genetic medicine and a renewed interest in studying how environmental factors, lifestyle choices, and attitudes affect people's health.

The takeaway, again and again, has been this: you must treat the whole patient. Laboratory values and imaging results are not sufficient to tell you what the patient is experiencing or what is influencing their outcomes. And why would we want to practice medicine in a world where humans could be reduced to sets of metrics on a spreadsheet?

Doctors in the Soviet Union experienced burnout due to heavy paperwork and an overwhelming number of patients, much like their counterparts in the U.S. today. Despite this, doctors can prioritize the well-being of patients over financial gain. I am pleased to see Dr. Torres sharing stories highlighting the importance of the doctor-patient relationship with readers today.

At my clinic, I take a patient-centered approach to medicine, which begins with actively listening to my patients. I allow them to express themselves entirely as long as it relates to their health. This is crucial because almost half of an accurate diagnosis comes from a patient's medical history. Surprisingly, today most doctors interrupt patients within 18 seconds on average, despite being taught in medical school about the importance of listening.

Palpation is my next step in the patient's examination process, which involves using my hands to examine the patient physically. I ensure that I never dismiss any pain during this process. Even when administering treatment, I regularly check and re-check the patient's pain levels. This process can be time-consuming, and initial visits can take two to two and a half hours. This is why my practice has only one exam room: I focus my attention on one patient at a time.

Many modern doctors consider this an unbelievable way to practice medicine. In some ways, I am lucky because of my relative independence from the hospital system. I am not subject to an administrator telling me how many patients I must see or what procedures I must prescribe to meet the hospital's financial goals. However, all doctors, regardless of their specialty or place of practice, can learn from Dr. Torres' approach and my own experience.

Medicine has been an integral part of society for a long time. Over the years, I have witnessed a significant shift in how medical technology has evolved, from black-and-white X-rays to high-resolution MRIs. I have seen a remarkable improvement in our care standards and understanding of the human mind and body. Our progress in medicine has been going strong for a while.

"The human factor", however, is a crucial aspect that cannot be measured by lab tests or genetic information. I'm motivated by the personal connections and impact I make on patients' lives, as well as their impact on mine. We are all human.

Scientific papers often try to eliminate human complications and focus on studying a large group of people while ignoring or removing the "confounding variables." This approach is effective in isolating variables and learning what each one does. However, when it comes to medicine, it is essential to treat an individual patient rather than just focusing on general trends.

Dr. Torres and I have worked together for 27 years and shared many patients during this time. We first met at a conference, where he expressed interest in my approach to treating patients. Dr. Torres has always been eager to find new ways to help his patients, and he was impressed by my approach to patient care. I, in turn, have been impressed by his dedication and skill in helping his patients. I now receive my injections for chronic pain from him.

Upon reading this compelling book, medical professionals and patients will develop a profound understanding of the essential nature of interpersonal connections in medicine and how human interactions impact the success of treatment and patients' overall well-being.

Dr. Felix Linetsky is a world-renowned leader in musculoskeletal pain. He is credited with coining the term "regenerative injection therapy" (RIT) to describe minimally invasive procedures, such as prolotherapy, to stimulate the healing process. He has received numerous awards for quality of patient care and published nearly two dozen articles and book chapters on the use of RIT in pain management. The Florida Academy of Pain Medicine created the Felix Linetsky Award for Excellence in Education in his honor.

Introduction

I have been practicing medicine for over 30 years and writing books for more than 10. At first, I confined myself to writing nonfiction books about medical topics or my life outside of work, but the COVID-19 pandemic dislodged something new in me. After a profoundly unsettling patient encounter during that time, which you'll read about in the first essay here, it was as though a floodgate had opened.

Essays about what it is like to practice medicine as a doctor and a human began pouring out. To my surprise, my colleagues in the medical community expressed gratitude for my bringing attention to the human side of medicine and articulating many experiences and emotions they had not seen discussed in medical education texts. KevinMD and Doximity were willing to give my essays a platform, enabling them to spark discussions among the thousands of doctors and healthcare workers who read these platforms.

As I wrote about my more personal experiences with patients I found that one thing about medicine was paramount to me: the human element. It was not the rare diagnoses or the tough clinical cases I solved that demanded expression. It was the quiet moments I had alone with patients in the clinic, in the hospital room, or over video chat that were the most meaningful moments to me—the reason I became a doctor.

I was surprised by the response the physician community had to my essays. So many readers voiced that they had had similar thoughts and feelings but had never heard them expressed in writing. A few others expressed strong negative feelings about my observations, triggering intense but needed conversations. It seemed that there was a great deal of thought and feeling around these questions of what it means to be both a human and a doctor in the 21st century, which was often going un-expressed amid the medical community's fervor for measurable, empirical facts, and reproducible experiments.

As my career advances, I have been reflecting on this increasing standardization and what sometimes seems to be a dehumanization of medicine in the United States. While I believe technology has the potential to help us bring humanity back to the forefront of medical practice while also improving diagnosis and care, I feel much of the human element has been lost since my early days of residency. This I would like to preserve in memory.

I was required to study the humanities, history, and philosophy in medical school. These books and classes heavily influenced my thinking about medicine. They asked questions like, "What is well-being, really?" "How do humans face death?" and "What is our relationship and our responsibility to our fellow humans?"

Today more than ever, I believe young doctors would benefit from the great works of literature and philosophy. In the face of a growing body of technical knowledge and increasingly stringent education funding environments, they are often given no incentive or opportunity to study the humanities and the liberal arts. They are exceedingly good at performing procedures and interpreting lab values and are often familiar with biochemical pathways that were unknown to science when I first practiced medicine. But I see them suffering when it comes to the human art of medicine.

What training they are given on how to talk to patients, break bad news, and how to support the whole person seems perfunctory. These young doctors have been taught in such great detail their obligations to standard reference ranges, clinical best practices, and metrics of success that machines can measure. They seem less certain about what they can afford to spare in terms of time and energy, to listen to patients, and take patients' individual wishes into account. Some seem to struggle with their sense of purpose, especially in an environment that often pressures them to take considerations other than patient relationships into account in their daily decisions.

I hope improvement is on the horizon with the advancement of Artificial Intelligence, which is already being used in some instances to read radiological scans before being manually reviewed and approved by radiologists. If used properly, I believe such technology could ease the burden of memorizing infinite facts and figures and allow future doctors to focus on stewardship of the patient as a human being in a human patient-doctor relationship.

But we aren't there yet. It is my belief that we all must vigilantly guard the human side of medicine, which is unlikely to speak for itself in meetings about time metrics, budgetary efficiency, and treatment decision algorithms.

Among the older school of doctors, there are those who believe in the primary importance of the physical exam. The art of examining patients fully requires physical touch and perceptive, individual attention. It is probably an empirically superior way of gathering comprehensive information about a patient's whole-person health status compared to the cursory touch-free 15-minute visits often encouraged in health systems today.

This degree of physical contact and attention to the patient actually does improve healing outcomes. This is not a totally superstitious idea; we now know that healing and growth are strongly affected by stress hormone levels, and that social support, skin-to-skin contact, and a patient's belief that they are being healed can create biochemical changes conducive to healing.

I have observed that, for better or worse, I can often predict which of my patients will recover and which will spiral downward based on their first visits to my clinic. It is the ones who trust me and feel safe with me who, very often, make full recoveries. I do not believe this is an accident.

As such, I urge all of us, doctors and patients alike, to defend medicine as a humanizing art in the years to come. While empirical research and double-blind controlled studies are things of true wonder and awe, patients are complex systems. We cannot treat patients like a mere set of numbers and be truly successful at optimizing their outcomes if we do not understand their stressors, environment, the actions that affect their health, and the drivers of those actions.

We owe it to ourselves and our patients to preserve the humanizing art of medicine. Let us begin a series of meditations on the human situations I have encountered in the clinic.

The Early Days of Telemedicine

Early in the pandemic, treating patients via video conference was new. I had "treated" patients via phone before when they could not find a qualified specialist in their area. Usually, this was to the dismay of my colleagues, who feared that I could not treat the patient properly without a physical exam. However, being *told* to use telemedicine as a matter of protocol and having video chat available recalibrated the dynamics.

The first patient I treated via video conference plunged me into the deep end of how telemedicine could change patient-doctor relationships, for better or worse. Speaking to this patient in his home instead of in the safety of my office left me so profoundly unsettled that I wrote my first-ever essay about the human experience of being a doctor to help cope with it.

This experience forced me to re-think how much I knew about my patients and how much power I had over their well-being. I am glad that I could share it in writing, and it must have resonated with many doctors because this first essay became the recipient of the Doximity OpMed Award for the highly charged summer of 2020.

Telemedicine Does Not Absolve Us as Doctors

As a pain management doctor, I routinely use the undefined to evaluate depressive symptoms in patients suffering from chronic pain. Typically, we furnish the patient with the questionnaire while they are waiting inside the examination room, and the patient fills out the form before ever seeing a physician. Once I'm in the room with the patient, I go over any areas for concern.

Telehealth appointments work differently. To avoid having to scan and send sensitive medical information by email, I go over the assessment questions orally with the patient at the outset of every appointment. That's what I was doing with Mr. McLeary when he got a bright idea.

Mr. McLeary is a man in his 60s who lives alone in a mobile home park. He has no immediate family and very few friends, but that is how he likes it. He describes himself as a germaphobe and a loner, uninterested in meeting new people. He boasts of his independence, but he neglects his physical health, often ignoring my prescriptions for regular exercise and proper nutrition.

I started our appointment by asking the depression inventory questions. When I arrived at a question about whether or not Mr. McLeary had ever entertained thoughts of suicide, he furrowed his brow for a moment and turned away from the camera. I could hear him rooting around in a nearby drawer. To my dismay, he reemerged, holding a pistol.

Two weeks before the appointment, we had received word from our clinic administrators that the office would have to shut down in light of COVID-19.

"No patient visits until further notice," our office manager said. She was heartbroken to have to let go scores of our staff members. The future was uncertain. Still, I felt we had an obligation to continue treating patients — which is where telemedicine came into play.

Several years ago, as the director of an anti-aging medical practice, I had contemplated offering concierge-style visits using remote technology. My team and I studied the possibility carefully, but in the end, the legal risks and liabilities outweighed the potential benefits. COVID-19 changed the calculus. We no longer had the luxury of requiring patients to walk in through the door.

I'm a physiatrist, and our chronically ill patients needed regular treatment. They depended on the timely delivery of pain prescriptions, especially when warding off potentially catastrophic withdrawal events. And, luckily for our clinic, Medicare had already recognized the issue and temporarily loosened telemedicine requirements during the pandemic. Thanks to a crack IT team, we signed up with a telehealth portal and began daily virtual appointments.

The first week went smoothly, marred only by a smattering of your typical technical glitches. Overall, I enjoyed the convenience of talking to and observing patients from the comfort of their homes. It felt almost like hopping on a video chat with friends and family. I had time to review patient medical histories without feeling rushed to dash off to another exam room. I was focused exclusively on the responses to my questions, and I was fully immersed in my patients' well-being. In turn, the patients appeared more comfortable, at ease, unhurried.

The new arrangement came with anthropological benefits as well. I cued into the patient's surroundings. I noticed the color of the walls and the decorations. I spotted potentially hazardous household obstacles, gathering exponentially more knowledge about living conditions than I ever had in the office. But, I was ill-prepared for Mr. McLeary.

"Doc," he said, wielding the pistol. "I might be an old man, but I've got my means."

He continued, telling me about how he had been traveling the world since he was in his early 20s. "I was in Turkey during the '70s and all that mess over there. I saw the death squads murdering people in the streets," he explained, referring to right-wing ultranationalists of the time. "I learned you have always got to have a gun for self-defense." Then, Mr. McLeary paused. My jaw gaped wide open as he added, "I suppose I could answer your question by pointing this pistol up to my temple and blowing my brains out while you watch."

He twisted the barrel up near his forehead.

"I will not do that, doc," he said, lowering the firearm to the desk. "I have thought about it in the past. I will admit that. But I am not suicidal, and I've got no intention to end things today. If I ever become a burden to other people," he said, caressing the pistol, "well, then I might reevaluate."

My heart pounded against my chest. I was powerless to intervene. Mr. McLeary could probably tell I was nervous. When I asked him politely to please put the pistol away, he replaced it inside the drawer. I barely made it through the rest of the appointment.

Our insurance malpractice carrier sends me what seems like weekly updates about telemedicine's pitfalls and how easy it is to get sued for what happens on a call. Still, no one had told me what to do when a patient turns suicidal — in your line of sight but at a distance. I am accustomed to rendering aid and comfort in the exam room. What was I supposed to do over a video call?

In hindsight, Mr. McLeary taught me a valuable lesson, even if his teaching style leaves much to be desired. Telemedicine does not absolve us as doctors from the very human aspects of our patient interactions. Since that bizarre encounter with Mr. McLeary, I have made some changes.

I start each call by asking for a physical address that I can use in case I need to send help. Also, I have established a direct emergency access line to contact my assistant. Finally, I always request an alternate phone number, preferably from someone close to the patient that I might enlist quickly if necessary. Thankfully, I did not have to use these safety measures in Mr. McLeary's case, but I am glad I have them at my disposal now.

When Textbooks Are Not Enough

My second essay on the experience of being a doctor was also wrenched from me by a profoundly troubling incident. In this case, it was the death of my mother—a death my intuition had expected but my rational mind ignored.

Throughout my medical school training, I was taught to think about numbers and probabilities. We were supposed to use textbooks, not our guts, to determine how likely any given patient was to suffer from a particular condition. We were taught to believe that the numbers were sacrosanct and unquestionable.

Yet this was always an incomplete view. The further modern medicine advances, the more we realize how many factors affect patient outcomes. Many of the factors we try to measure and control for today were not even known to science when I first started practicing medicine in the 1990s. Could some doctors have had an intuition that unseen factors made some patients different from others before the data discovered previously unknown genetic traits?

How often might our intuition see things that the numbers in the textbooks are not yet advanced enough to understand?

My connection with my mother was one of the most critical relationships of my life. Losing her to a complication she *should* have been low-risk for deeply affected the way I practice medicine today—especially since, according to the numbers, it shouldn't have happened.

Ever since her death, I have encouraged my fellow physicians to trust their guts above the numbers in the textbooks when their guts are trying to send a clear message. My essay about the power of intuition in clinical decision-making first appeared in Doximity OpMed in July of 2022.

Why We Should Pay More Attention To Our Intuition

My mother died almost two decades ago. She was only 69 years old and perfectly healthy. Still today, I wonder if I—as a physician and as a son—could have done more to save her life.

When my mom first fell on the kitchen floor, shattering her hip, she called and begged me for help. We got her to the hospital, and I arranged for a surgeon I trusted to operate on her. After an open-reduction and internal fixation, she moved to a rehabilitation center. She was frustrated by the loss of mobility and independence, but she was dogged in her daily exercises, making rapid progress toward a swift discharge. Suddenly, it all came crashing down.

She had pushed herself too hard and fractured her hip a second time. The setback was devastating. We had to prepare her for surgery once again.

I cannot forget the last few nights I spent with her at the hospital. She was serene in some ways, but she was also terrified. She had suffered from anxiety her entire life, and this situation made everything worse. I reassured her. I was keeping tabs on everything.

Still, I hid from her my lingering fear: blood clots. I had an intuition, but I silenced it. Her doctors were monitoring for complications. I convinced myself I had no business stepping in at that point.

And then it happened. My mother felt a pain in her chest, which she thought was simply a panic attack. She begged for her anxiety medication one minute, and the next minute she was gone. I couldn't intervene.

I have never felt so helpless as a physician or as a human being.

After 30 years of practicing medicine, I can freely admit that many of my clinical decisions are rooted in my intuition, buttressed by my thousands of past experiences and a reservoir of subconscious knowledge. But intuition is more than just experience or expertise. My experience with my mother begs the question to this day: Where are the limits of analytical thought, and how should our intuition take charge?

Our modern world owes many of its luxuries to the scientific method — an empirical approach to decision-making in various walks of life. Is there a cost, though, to this fanatical reliance on what we can see and prove? Are we too reluctant to discuss the role intuition plays in the clinical setting?

There is an intuitive urge inside us, particularly among those who practice the medical arts. It's a powerful aspect of the human spirit, and I don't think we should just ignore it when it comes to providing care.

Does that mean we should ignore the cold hard facts in front of us? No. Should we cast aside probabilities and decision matrices? No. I'm advocating for nuance — that is to say, if you have an intuition about a patient's care, you should indulge it. That's what separates a human medical doctor from a machine or an algorithm.

Of course, we can't confuse intuition with fear. You may feel uneasy before embarking on a new adventure, and it may seem as though your intuition is directing you to hold fast. But fear is physiological. It is anxiety produced by chemicals in our brains, triggered by the prospect of the unknown.

Intuition is far more psychological than that. The only way to really tell the difference in practice, I have learned, is through deep introspection. Personally, I try to meditate on my intuitions before diving fully into the project of exploring them.

With this methodology, I can explore my body and discern the evolutionary safeguards present in things like fear and anxiety from the blessing of intuition. I aim to discover whether my instincts lead me to expand or contract in every situation.

I don't know for sure whether it was a blood clot that finally killed my mother. The more I read about so-called "undefined," the more I question whether that might not have caused death. I have learned something from experience, whatever the scientific explanation: I should never just ignore my intuition. These days, I apply that lesson daily in my medical practice.

My patients are not science experiments. My care cannot be reduced solely to a rote process of trial and error based entirely on probabilities derived from de-personalized studies. I have to be rigorous about the scientific basis for my medical decisions. Still, I am equally committed to exploring that feeling I get, that instinct to test an unusual theory from time to time. We shouldn't leave our intuitions out of our decisions.

WHEN THE DOCTOR UNDERSTANDS MORE THAN YOU KNOW

O ver the years, I have had patients ask to see a different doctor. The reasons are usually merely annoying, but this one was heartbreaking.

I understood this patient's case better than she ever could have imagined because of my lifelong struggles with weight and body image. I spent the first 40 years of my life being ashamed of my body, trying to hide it and avert attention from myself. So to hear that this patient had believed I would judge her for her weight was heartbreaking for me.

In today's medical system, too many patients report feeling that their doctors are judging them or even making false assumptions about their lifestyles based on their physical characteristics. Overweight patients report that doctors often seem to blame any symptoms they have on their weight. At the same time, women continue to feel that many doctors dismiss their symptoms as "female troubles" or medical anxiety, even when they turn out to have a severe medical condition.

My first hand understanding of this woman's fear of being judged led me to write this essay, first published in KevinMD in July 2022.

The Importance of Non-Judgmental Empathy

It has always been difficult for medical professionals to balance the time needed for personal care, both physical and emotional, against the overwhelming demands of their time. This is particularly true today, given the extraordinary pressures created by health challenges generated through external factors, such as the pandemic and those caused by genetics or lifestyle choices. However, focusing on this balance is critical for the welfare of both the doctors and the patients.

A few months ago, a woman called my office's nursing staff to request a physician change for her upcoming appointment. The request wasn't odd, as patients ask to be seen by a different doctor for many reasons. However, in this case, the patient was not asking for a different doctor because they wanted a different opinion, a lack of trust, or other similar reasons. In the past, patients had even requested a change for such a simple reason as not relating to my accent. This has happened more than once! However, the woman wanted a "less fit" doctor in this case.

I must admit that I found this request strange, but it made me think. I assume her rationale was that I wouldn't be sympathetic to her condition or life choices. She was in her fifties and had a "broken body." I wouldn't be able to relate. Perhaps a doctor with more average health status and body shape would approach the problem with less rigor or intensity.

I've never recommended a specialist based on their physical appearance and would not expect anyone else to do so. I have always believed that a healthy doctor would project more credibility and authority. I hadn't considered this intimidating. Perhaps it wasn't the outward appearance but the idea that I would have less empathy for her situation.

As I thought about these possibilities, I asked myself how I could use this reaction to improve my physician practice. This wasn't the first time I've considered how a physician's lifestyle might affect their patients. For instance, it is patently contradictory when an overweight medical provider recommends diet and exercise. I can imagine patients asking themselves, why should they alter their comfort zone if something is not important enough for their doctor? The same advice from a fit doctor might elicit some level of cynicism in thinking that somehow being healthy comes naturally or easily.

In principle, I would like to motivate my patients and help wean them from the excuses and thinking that keep many of them in an unhealthy state. I want to challenge them to change and improve through better life choices. How does a doctor do that while still relating and keeping in the forefront the particular challenges of every patient? I certainly do not want to demotivate through appearance or demeanor.

I have written books on my voyage to better health through exercise and nutrition. There are books in my office. The content and cover of these books articulate a process of transformation. Both cover and content show a vulnerable and candid story of a doctor having issues with weight and self-esteem and the process of recovery once the realization set in that, without change, there would be severe health consequences. This possibility is available to both doctors and patients.

The intent is not for everyone to achieve a competition-level athletic build but to find more enjoyment in life through better health. This is true of both doctors and patients. Everyone has individual roadblocks to achieving this. For each patient, the reasons are too many to count. For doctors, it is primarily a lack of time, overwhelming stress, and emotional overload. It is not a lack of understanding of the science. A balance must be achieved, and, to do that, first, we must understand the relevance and impact of this balance.

In medical school, I was trained to earn the trust of my patients. The rationale behind this was that patients follow and listen to doctors they trust. I always assumed I had to lead by example if I aspired to build that kind of trust with my patients.

My mantra has been that wellness and fitness are essential for good leadership. Furthermore, physician leadership is pivotal for excellent patient outcomes. Also, part of the very reason I engage in healthy practices is what I see every day when these are disregarded. The ravaging aftermath of being overweight, the medical conditions of lack of exercise, and poor and unhealthy eating.

Embracing a non-judgmental attitude reassures patients that they can seek medical guidance without fear of embarrassment or criticism, creating an indispensable part of a doctor's professionalism. Whether the doctor is fit or struggling with health issues, conveying information in this non-judgmental empathy elevates the conversation to both intent and science.

I think we all have an inclination—at least from time to time—to judge others. No matter how experienced, compassionate, and professional we are as physicians, we're still human. I can admit that I have indeed struggled with patients like the 65-year-old morbidly obese male who complains at every visit about how hard it is to control his blood sugar levels with the medications prescribed. I want to convince him so badly about diet and exercise, but I have tried, and often, these patients don't want to hear it. Pharmacological or surgical interventions are the preferred route for many.

I know I cannot magically change a patient's attitudes about their health. Nevertheless, I still believe that the best I can do for my patients is to offer them my sincere professional advice without prejudice or discrimination. If my physical presence is intimidating to some, I won't begrudge them for seeking a doctor who makes them feel more comfortable.

In the end, I still believe that leading by example is essential for a physician and that I can use my personal experience to inspire positive change. After all, I am here to help.

Toeing the Line as a Healthcare Provider

As a pain management specialist, I may have stronger feelings about obesity than most doctors. My book, *Epigenetics and the Psychology of Weight Loss*, features a chapter about a patient who I was sure would die soon when I first saw him.

After becoming nearly bedridden with chronic pain, he had gained weight and was maxing out the allowed portion of opiates. This was understandable; it was also tragic. I risked damaging his spine every time I gave him injections due to the difficulty in finding the correct location beneath his body fat, and I could not in good conscience recommend him for surgery, knowing that his weight put him at extremely high risk for respiratory arrest under anesthesia.

I candidly shared my fears about his weight's effect on him. I knew that this patient would likely never successfully tame his pain or recover any of his range of motion as long as he had so much weight straining the injured nerves and muscles of his back. I knew that his situation was likely to continue to get worse unless he could lose weight, relieving the strain of gravity placed upon his injury and placing him at lower-risk for pain management procedures.

This patient then blew me away with his dedication to fitness. Today, he has lost almost three-quarters of the weight he had when I first met him and is happily surprising his physical therapist by insisting that he wants to learn to ride his motorcycle again now that he is in his late 70s.

I am happy that we as a culture have mostly moved away from the 1990s when being pathologically emaciated was often considered the beauty standard. But we cannot ignore that the other extreme is just as dangerous: excess body fat does make many medical conditions more painful and more dangerous.

For this reason, we must be responsible care providers. We must never assume that a patient's symptoms are caused *only* by their weight, but we must also be honest with those whose lives are worsened or shortened by excess body fat.

This essay was first published in KevinMD in September of 2022.

ARE WE TOO SCARED TO TALK TO OUR PATIENTS ABOUT THEIR WEIGHT?

Talking about weight isn't easy. Case in point, I was scheduled to perform five back-to-back fluoroscopically guided procedures. This was not unusual, but all my scheduled patients happened to be seriously overweight. Excess fat and skin made it difficult to see my needles during the interventional procedures. Therefore, what was ordinarily a routine procedure suddenly became complex and challenging.

I am an interventional pain management physician. For many of my patients, the underlying cause of their medical conditions or a major contributing factor is their obesity. When I encounter these overweight patients, my first instinct is to want to counsel them about nutrition and wellness. I want to warn them that their excess weight could lead to premature death and lower quality of life. I instinctively want to explain to them that the procedures they are asking me to complete are likely to be more challenging and riskier due to their obesity.

Of course, it is not that simple and shouldn't be. For one, I am not comfortable being blunt with patients about weight problems. I always want to be sensitive to how excess weight makes people feel. In most cases, it is natural to communicate with a patient using accepted medical terms. However, when you are trying to focus on the person and not just the condition, terms like obesity can be offensive and be received with many unintended connotations.

Our society can be cruel at times with this issue. I have been overweight and suffered a lot of pain and anxiety, including bullying. I want to avoid causing my patients any pain. This requires removing some of the directness of orthodox clinical terms with language that will be better received.

Nevertheless, on the other hand, are we missing an opportunity to help by failing to be direct? Do we owe our patients a sense of urgency around this topic? In not addressing this condition head-on, why do we avoid this specific medical issue when delivering care?

Interestingly, there are other behaviors — aggravated conditions, such as smoking and lung disease — where it seems easier to approach patients with much more bluntness. Again, this difference seems to be ingrained in societal perceptions and judgments. The psychological backdrop is particularly relevant in dealing with this topic.

Most people do not lose weight to make medical procedures easier for their doctors. The media promotes losing weight principally around the allure of vanity: e.g., slim, beautiful models. In modern society, overall health is a secondary benefit to weight loss.

Correctly promoting a healthy self-image has, at times, the unintended consequence that remaining in an unhealthy weight condition is OK. Messaging that promotes complacency in this area under the guise of self-acceptance may exacerbate our societal crises created by excess weight and unhealthy eating habits.

Hopefully, focusing more on comprehensive studies describing the disastrous health consequences of obesity may motivate more people to achieve and maintain appropriate body weight for the right reason. Still, conscious dieters who are already aware that the real purpose of losing weight is to promote health and longevity may become frustrated when they have difficulty shedding those extra pounds.

With little to no success, yo-yo dieting becomes a part of their lives as they try various diets. It is incumbent on doctors involved in their care to discern between obese patients trying to address their condition but having a challenging time from those that choose to disregard or misunderstand the consequences of long-term obesity. Both attitudes should be addressed but in fundamentally different ways. Directness may have a larger role to play in the latter.

Most people do not understand that obesity is often a symptom of an underlying condition, physical or psychological. This includes many who work in the health community. At times, an approach to recommend losing weight with a health focus as a primary aim may be placing the cart before the horse. A weight problem's origin or root cause must be ascertained and dealt with first.

For instance, obese people are less likely to exercise than those already within their target weight. Understanding and addressing each patient's lack of motivation is essential. Every person is different. As mentioned earlier, the physical fitness level of the metabolic-healthy obese patient versus the physical fitness status of the metabolic-unhealthy obese patient needs to be considered before drawing any conclusions or recommending a course of action. Studies show that you do not need to be thin to reap the health benefits of exercise. Based on my experience with wellness patients, waist circumference matters the most.

As mentioned earlier, a slim waistline protects you against diabetes and heart disease. Being overweight can feel awful, especially in modern society.

For some, it can be the worst thing imaginable. It can immobilize the individual, both physically and emotionally.

The emotional reactions can be disproportionate and perpetuate the vicious cycle of poor physical activity and weight gain, leading to poor health. Many of these poor health consequences associated with obesity involve higher risks during medical procedures. Given the objective and scientific consequences of obesity, I would argue that there is a need to change our conversations with obese patients.

There will always be an expectation to show sensitivity, empathy, and caring. But there is also a need to ensure that conversations are clear, unequivocal, and direct in understanding what is at stake concerning short-term and long-term health, longevity, and overall quality of life. Over-focusing on the potential adverse reaction to the message is not fair to the patient and is a dereliction of duty.

Fostering a caring and strong relationship with each patient and credibility through the consistency of messaging will always help deliver "tough love" medical advice. Each patient is unique and, therefore, should be treated accordingly. This aspect of medical practice represents more art than science and is a skill worth developing.

WHEN NUTRITION AND PSYCHOLOGY COLLIDE

In my 2022 book *Epigenetics and the Psychology of Weight Loss*, I discuss how obesity and caloric excess can negatively affect human health and how winning the battle against poor nutrition is often as much a psychological battle as a battle of knowledge or material resources. After all, as I often hear from my patients, "I know what I should be eating. I can't convince myself to do it."

In my practice, I get an especially acute look at the negative impact that poor nutrition can have on both obesity and pain. Some of the procedures I must perform and some of the medications I must prescribe to patients to relieve their pain can have life-threatening complications when obesity is present. In addition, a growing body of research shows that chemical messengers derived from our foods can improve or worsen the pain processes of our nervous systems.

This has led to my philosophy of focusing on nutrition first. While weight loss may be a necessary goal for some patients if they wish to experience pain relief and increased longevity, the root cause of both obesity and some forms of pain and inflammation can be nutrition.

The book itself takes the reader on a journey from the African savannas, where hunter-gatherers still live and eat in traditional ways, to my patient, Jim, who defied all medical expectations when he lost most of his body weight and returned to an active, healthy lifestyle in his 70s after a decade of debilitating chronic pain complicated by obesity.

However, for this excerpt, which KevinMD published in October of 2022, I focus on how obesity and chronic pain can form a self-perpetuating cycle that requires an understanding of psychology to escape.

WE CANNOT IGNORE NUTRITION'S IMPACT ON BOTH PAIN AND OBESITY

We know that people with chronic pain are more likely to be obese; but does this happen because people with chronic pain struggle to exercise and suffer from a high load of stress hormones which promote stress eating, or does it happen because obesity causes more wear and tear on joints, which can lead to back problems, pinched nerves, and challenges to exercise? Or could it be that both scenarios are sometimes true?

This question affects our decision-making as doctors in a big way. When we see a patient who is overweight and in pain, what do we tackle first? Do we assume that the extra weight is responsible for the pain? Or do we assume that the pain must be resolved before more exercise and nutrient-dense dietary choices become feasible?

In recent years, physicians are thankfully more aware of the dangers of "fatphobia"—a prejudice against fat people which can lead some doctors to incorrectly assume that the patient's weight is the cause of any health problems they may report.

Tragically, fatphobia is believed to contribute to higher morbidity and mortality rates for fat patients since some doctors may fail to order potentially lifesaving diagnostic tests for fat patients due to an assumption that a person's body weight must be the cause of their symptoms.

A wide variety of illnesses, including heart attacks and cancer, have been missed in their earliest and most treatable stages as a result of doctors assuming that symptoms like pain, shortness of breath, and overall feelings of illness and discomfort were related to patients' high body mass index. As doctors, we must treat all patients equally and avoid unwarranted assumptions about our patient's health.

However, there is also evidence that patients with high BMIs have worse outcomes from many health problems,[1] and several other important causes of morbidity and mortality.

So, let us look at the evidence for which comes first: obesity or chronic pain.

Early evidence may suggest that obesity aggravates chronic pain.[2] One well-known 1992 study showed that women with osteoarthritis experienced less pain after losing weight;[3] another study in 2004 showed that weight loss in obese women reduced pain levels and allowed the women in the study to undertake a broader range of daily activities. A 2015 study found that obesity increases chronic pain, and chronic pain also tends to

---

1. Demeulemeester, F., de Punder, K., van Heijningen, M., & van Doesburg, F. (2021). Obesity as a risk factor for severe COVID-19 and complications: A Review. *Cells, 10*(4), 933. https://doi.org/10.3390/cells10040933

increase weight through reduced levels of physical activity and increased stress eating.[4]

According to Stone and Broderick's, there appears to be a linear relationship between chronic pain and body mass index (BMI).[5] McVinnie's goes on to elaborate that obesity's impact on pain may be explained by the increased levels of inflammatory markers interleukin 6 (IL-6), tumor necrosis factor α (TNF- α), and C-reactive protein (CRP).[6] All of these are chemical messengers that change the body's metabolic function, and all are found at higher levels, on average, in obese patients.

More investigation is needed into why this occurs and whether this relation is caused directly by a person's BMI or by matters like dietary choices, which may be correlated to (but not caused by) both obesity and higher levels of these chemical messengers. Since some chemical messengers are known to increase in response to different types of foods, illnesses, and stresses, there is more work about correlation vs. causation.

---

4. Okifuji A, Hare BD. The association between chronic pain and obesity. J Pain Res. 2015 Jul 14;8:399-408. doi: 10.2147/JPR.S55598. PMID: 26203274; PMCID: PMC4508090.

5. Stone AA, Broderick JE. Obesity and pain are associated in the United States. Obesity (Silver Spring). 2012 Jul;20(7):1491-5. doi: 10.1038/oby.2011.397. Epub 2012 Jan 19. Erratum in: Obesity (Silver Spring). 2012 Jul;20(7):1546. PMID: 22262163.

6. McVinnie DS. Obesity and pain. Br J Pain. 2013 Nov;7(4):163-70. doi: 10.1177/2049463713484296. PMID: 26516520; PMCID: PMC4590160.

However, the fact remains that a robust correlation was found between a person's BMI and their levels of chronic pain. It is reasonable to assume, then, that lifestyle changes which lead to weight loss should also lead to reductions in chronic pain.

Another possible mechanism by which obesity may aggravate or even cause chronic pain is the simple mechanical stress placed on joints when carrying extra weight. We know that proteins called "mechanoreceptors," which detect mechanical loads on the cartilage that cushions our bones at the joints, are activated when our joints are asked to carry heavy loads.

This activation of mechanoreceptors in our cartilage leads to the activation of intracellular pathways that produce metalloproteases and interleukin 1 (IL-1). These enzymes and chemical messengers degrade the cartilage extracellular matrix and activate inflammatory processes, which can lead to sensations of pain and illness.

This all makes intuitive sense. In obese patients, the joints and circulatory system are asked to handle a significantly heavier workload than the body systems of other people.

In highly fit people, this may be less of a problem; a person with strong supporting muscles and a highly trained cardiovascular system may be prepared to handle this workload without health problems. This is illustrated by several overweight athletes and performers, who achieve astonishing athleticism, which is all the more astonishing for being performed while carrying considerably more weight on their bones, muscles, and joints than most people.

However, a person with poor nutrition and an inactive lifestyle has not developed their body's capabilities to be able to handle this load, and the combination of poor fitness and nutrition with a high workload placed on the body by a high body mass is likely to result in illness and injury over time.

However, it is essential to know that body weight is not the whole story of chronic pain. Many people who are not overweight struggle with chronic pain. While studies suggest that a decrease usually follows weight loss in chronic pain, it may not eliminate it. Nor is obesity necessarily the first cause of chronic pain; sometimes, it is a consequence of reduced mobility from chronic pain, albeit a consequence that usually worsens the chronic pain.

We cannot neglect chronic pain issues regarding weight loss programs and exercise. Pain is painful. That sounds obvious, but when we are in pain, the initial reaction is to remove the pain-causing stimulus. If walking causes pain, we stop walking. It is a natural survival mechanism. Moreover, when pain is caused by tissue damage from mechanical overloading of weight on our joints, sometimes that is a wise course of action.

According to McVinnie (2013), a study investigating activity levels in patients with knee osteoarthritis found that 12.9 percent of males and 7.7 percent of females were reaching only the minimum recommended amount of physical activity. Activity levels are unlikely to rise significantly as long as they are hampered by chronic pain.

Additionally, we cannot ignore nutrition's impact on both pain and obesity. Pleasure eating is a real issue, especially in those with pain. We know that stress hormones encourage people to eat more fatty and high-carb foods while discouraging the consumption of nutrient-dense low-calorie foods. Eating is used both as a mechanism to help cope with pain and as an analgesic to reduce pain temporarily.

Both pain and obesity can have a multitude of causes. Therefore, reducing pain and body weight should be approached in a multifactorial way; nutritionally, physically, mentally, and emotionally. Failure to do so may result in short-term success but long-term failure.

ARE WE LISTENING?

I was shocked recently to read a statistic about how often doctors interrupt patients when they are speaking. According to one study, the median time until a patient who spoke was interrupted by a doctor was 18 seconds. Patients had to speak less than that to avoid being interrupted by their doctor.

The study's authors astutely point out that this seemingly low tolerance for patients expressing their thoughts, feelings, and experiences may contribute to patient noncompliance and distrust of physicians. When patients feel that doctors and the medical establishment are uninterested in their thoughts and feelings, it is natural that they would feel disengaged or even averse to following doctors' advice.

This is another reason why preserving medicine as a humanizing art is essential. Many misdiagnoses and poor treatment decisions can be traced to doctors who cut patients off without getting the whole story about their lives or their symptoms.

I had my own experience of realizing I had failed to listen to a patient a few years back. While this story fortunately has a happy ending, it could have ended much differently if not for the patient's religious beliefs about self-harm. I always remember this memory as a reminder to listen to my patients' words and behaviors.

KevinMD first published this essay in November of 2022.

Not Listening Carefully to a Vulnerable Patient Can Become a Matter of Life or Death

Paula came to my office on a Monday afternoon, a few months after burying her husband. She and John had been inseparable. They were both my patients, so I knew John had spent the last six months battling lung cancer. They had been married forty-five years when John died. I sincerely offered Paula my condolences on that Monday afternoon. I could tell she was in pain and shared how she missed John terribly.

When Paula came in for a follow-up appointment sometime later, I happened to be short on time that day. I had a full schedule of patients to see. As usual, I was tired, in my mid-career focus to keep the practice afloat. I was polite but a little condescending when she told me she was planning to run a marathon to honor John's memory. I didn't take much notice when she shared her intentions. I figured they were just that, intentions that would not materialize.

It was natural to feel skeptical. Paula had never run before in her life. She really never exerted herself physically much at all. Cynically, I didn't think there was any chance she would make it. Then in my forties, I could not imagine that a woman over sixty could suddenly find her passion for exercise and running, particularly in a full-length marathon.

A few months passed before I heard from Paula again. She looked youthful, reinvigorated. She had finished a marathon. In fact, she was running all the time now. And though it is a story of personal success over grief, it is not.

After telling me about her marathon, Paula suddenly paused and became serious. And then she shared the surprising fact that she didn't really run to honor her husband's memory. When John died, she was determined to run a marathon as a way of killing herself by exerting herself beyond her tolerance.

Paula had grown severely depressed after her husband's death. She was suicidal. But she'd grown up religious, and frankly, she was scared to kill herself in a violent way. She thought if she just pushed herself too hard physically, without any training, her body would give out, and she could end her life.

Regretfully, I realized that I had missed all the signs. Paula had come to me, her caregiver, and I had cavalierly brushed her aside because I was too busy and too tired to care. Of course, I had been polite and examined her joint pains, but I wasn't really listening to my patient. I couldn't see what she was going through, and I should have.

Nowadays, it is easy to get burned out as a physician. We absorb our patients' discomforts and fears. We rush from one appointment to the next, checking the boxes, too distracted to look beyond the chart. A patient's pain is more than the physical pain they report to us on a scale of one to ten.

In fact, often, patients we interact with each day are likely depressed. We might be the only person in their lives who have confidence in sharing their struggles. It is, in fact, a key part of our jobs to listen, to look out for them, and to offer our support.

Depression cuts away at humanity. It makes the person question the motivation for hanging on to life. Most times, hanging on is too difficult for those people who suffer from severe depression. In fact, the pain and symptoms of depression often make it difficult to ask for help, like in Paula's case.

In our medical profession, we must make time to listen to every patient and show empathy. Somehow, we must find the time to communicate the message that life is worth living and that there is a purpose in life, even when we lose a loved one.

We should try to see their sadness even as they try to hide it from us. Let's make sure we, as physicians and caregivers, take the necessary steps to recognize the signs and symptoms of depression to help our patients avoid becoming victims of that depressive state. It is critical and relevant that those patients we come into contact with daily, who struggle silently, can feel safe asking for help.

Thankfully, Paula didn't kill herself running a marathon without any training. She finished by sheer force of will and unexpectedly gave her new purpose. She continued running well into her seventies and got healthier and happier. But the fact remains that this story could have ended differently and tragically.

The nature of our work makes it easier at times to remain at a superficial level with our patients—to be polite without really being human. I think it is our duty to take the intentional approach and strive to really listen. We won't hear everything, of course, but there will be those times when we understand the real cry for help and make a difference.

The Power of Distance Healing

I had my first telemedicine patient in the early 1990s when video chat hadn't been invented yet. The patient was desperate: she had been physically examined by many doctors, but none in her geographic area had the specialized knowledge to diagnose her. Although there was a great deal of skepticism about treating a patient without having examined them, I had no choice but to try to do something for her.

Since then, we have seen telemedicine expand the ways in which patients can be treated. While I am a big believer in the human connection and even the power of the healing touch, I also believe in connecting patients to the best care for them regardless of where they live or their ability to travel. We must remember these two opposing considerations as we navigate the advancing world of telemedicine today.

I shared my reflection on the benefits and risks of telemedicine with KevinMD in January of 2023. Around that time, it became clear that telemedicine was not just a pandemic emergency measure but a place to stay.

How Technology is Transforming Medicine and Making Distance Healing a Reality

My first job as a "real" doctor was in 1991.

During one of those early days in my career, one of my coworkers — a woman who worked in reception — approached me for help. Even then, I could recognize a look of desperation. It reminded me of the look I saw in my sister when all she could do to lessen the pain she had suffered for so long was to slide ineffective sole inserts into her shoes. Later, she would be diagnosed with rheumatoid arthritis. It was the characteristic look of utter powerlessness.

It turned out that my coworker had not approached me about herself. Her mother, who lived in California then, suffered from extreme and chronic pain. I sympathized since I had felt the same sense of helplessness as my sister. Apparently, her mother had not been able to find successful help for her condition. So, I asked her to have her mother come in for some tests to see if I could do anything. However, she could not fly her out to Florida, where my practice was located.

My immediate inclination was to say that I couldn't do anything from three thousand miles away. But the thought of what my sister had gone through prior to her diagnosis prompted me to do otherwise. With some hesitation and misgivings, I agreed to "treat" her mother over the phone. I wanted to do something, even if it was just to listen to this woman's frustration and concerns over the phone.

The woman started to describe every aspect of her excruciating symptoms immediately from the moment we connected on the phone. In a strange way, I couldn't help feeling I was already treating her just by listening. She itemized the parade of physicians she had consulted in the past year. Emphatically, she lamented how not even one of them had made any difference when it came to mitigating the enormous pain she was suffering. I asked her if she had had a complete blood test panel and that, if not, she needed to have one done right away.

I carefully explained what areas in which to focus, such as the sedimentation rate in her blood. I explained in the simplest terms that the sedimentation rate in the blood, when elevated significantly, could be consistent with a diagnosis of polymyalgia rheumatica. Surprisingly, she seemed to receive my advice with excitement rather than concern. I have never heard anyone so overjoyed to learn they might have a disease!

The woman's test returned positive, and the rest, as they say, is history. The final chapter in her nearly two-year battle against debilitating pain began with a phone call and the stroke of a pen. The proper analyses and a correct diagnosis made all the difference.

There is no cure for polymyalgia rheumatica. Nevertheless, there are practical ways of detecting the disease in its early stages, managing its symptoms, and ultimately thriving, despite its onset, to enable a high quality of life with such a chronic disease.

When I spoke with my colleague's mother, the concept of telemedicine was not a consideration in standard medical care. It would have seemed ludicrous among certain medical opinions. The idea that a doctor could treat a patient without seeing them in person could have even been considered irresponsible.

As recently as the 2010s, most health care providers refused to offer telemedicine visits due to liability concerns. There was significant fear of being sued if a patient was unhappy with their results or if confidential health information somehow leaked because communications were being conducted via phone or video.

It took the COVID-19 pandemic to change this attitude when the concern of patients in person for medical care could place them in danger. This is a change that many patients have welcomed enthusiastically. Since 2020, the use of telemedicine has skyrocketed by a whopping 1,500 percent among Medicaid patients alone. Adopting change is difficult, and this transition to acceptance of a major approach to health care is astounding.

Many patients feel they have greater access to health care now that every doctor's visit does not necessarily involve physically traveling to a health care facility covered by their insurance during business hours. Patients with mobility challenges and those struggling with getting time off work, procuring childcare, or being unable to cover transportation costs have benefitted particularly.

I recently had a patient complain to me about the difficulty she was having in obtaining mental health treatment. The mental health providers covered by her insurance did not offer telemedicine, and the nearest office her insurance covered was a 40-minute commute from her home.

"I must take three hours out of my week for a one-hour therapist visit," she complained. "I do not know how I am supposed to do that on top of work and family responsibilities." Her previous insurance, she explained, had covered a therapist who offered telemedicine. As a result, she was able to have therapy sessions for just an hour per week at her home. Since changing insurance policies, she has not seen a therapist in eight months.

While every doctor knows there are cases where a patient needs to be seen in person to rule out life-threatening conditions, in practice, the vast majority of doctor's visits do not fall into this category.

Which would we rather have: patients being seen via a video call at the right time to be seen but where we cannot physically perform specific tests in real-time or not being seen by the appropriate care provider for a prolonged period because getting to the doctor is too challenging?

I don't pretend to say that the answer is straightforward. It isn't. But I am glad for this change in expanding the coverage available, particularly in light of the challenges to medical access in this country.

Likely, the answer will be found in further defining the proper use for telemedicine and the controls for its appropriate use to prevent over-reaches and abuse of this flexibility. Technological advances in communication, bio-analytics, digital biometrics, bio-scanning, and other innovations will make medicine at a distance feel less and less science fiction and more routine.

IF WE WANT CHANGE, WE MUST PAY ATTENTION TO OPPORTUNITIES

Decades ago, I was living with my wife in Puerto Rico when I saw a job ad for a doctor needed in the United States. This chance glance at a break room magazine would change my life and set me on an entirely new course.

I want to share this story because of the level of anxiety and frustration I see among new doctors regarding the resident matching program. Many young doctors are told that their futures will be determined by which institution, if anyone, they match with. Those who do not end up where they want to be with their match can feel like they have missed their window to create the lives they want.

This is not the case. Life is full of choices, especially for medical doctors whose services may be in demand anywhere in the world. Many unorthodox paths are available to doctors at any stage in their careers, some of which I describe in more detail later in this book.

This goes for doctors and members of the general public alike: if we want a change, we must remain open to the opportunities. Many opportunities for change fall into our laps regularly. Will we seize them?

My essay on how small decisions and the willingness to take a chance transformed my life path first appeared in KevinMD in January of 2023.

Why Taking Risks is Worth It: A Doctor's Journey from Uncertainty to Opportunity

There were no smartphones when I was a medical resident in the late 80s in Puerto Rico. During my last year, while waiting for a lecturer to arrive, I grabbed a medical journal from the conference room table to kill some time. I flipped through the pages, skimming the titles of the articles and looking at some of the advertisements. When I was about to put the journal down, I saw a small and straightforward announcement for a fellowship in Musculoskeletal Medicine in Louisiana at LSU Medical School, New Orleans.

I already had two small children and a job offer at the time. My parents and my in-laws were providing childcare. My wife, a pathologist, was finishing her own residency, and she already had a prestigious job offer she was eager to accept. I was content with my life and my future.

Or so I thought.

I had no urge to uproot my family and move to the States. Besides, my English needed a little (or a lot) of work. The pressures around practicing medicine—particularly as a new doctor—are overwhelming on a good day. I had much anxiety around the unknown, about testing my skill in a new place.

Still, out of curiosity, I inquired about the position.

Four months later, I was still waiting to receive a reply. I assumed LSU was working its way through a slew of better candidates. No harm, no foul, I thought. Then, one morning in early May of 1990, I received a letter offering an on-site interview in Louisiana.

Many of my classmates knew what they wanted from their careers. They knew where they were going. I had cobbled together a series of assignments and was just a few months away from graduating.

Despite intense fear, something told me to go for the interview. It was only my second time visiting the United States.

To my surprise, I was offered the position the same weekend as my interview. I accepted within forty-eight hours after discussing it with my wife. I made the decision based on a gut feeling that the opportunity needed seizing. Thirty-three years later, I am convinced I made the right decision. The fellowship created opportunities I could never have imagined for my wife and me.

When I think about my children and their lives, I can see how my choice has given them their own opportunities and privileges. Looking back, it seems like such an obvious choice, like it was meant to be. But how close did I come to not even applying?

Sometime after I began the fellowship, the program director confessed that I was not his first choice. The first choice, who had already signed a contract and committed to the program, decided to go elsewhere. That put the director in a bind. He would lose the fellowship money for his research if he did not have a fellow. Luckily for him, I applied out of the blue just in time.

In medical school and later in our residencies, we experience everything from hope to panic. Uncertainty is everywhere, and it causes stress. On match day, hundreds of medical students all over the country fear that this decision will dictate everything important about their future. Before that, college students worried that if they did not get into the right medical school, they would not have the career they had always dreamed of.

We should say more, especially in our profession, that no one thing is determinative. Too often, we focus on our desired outcome to the exclusion of all sorts of possibilities. If you decide where you are going and commit obsessively to getting there, you very well might find you are going nowhere.

The flighty fellow whose job I took in Louisiana ended up becoming a friend of mine. When he found out I was taking his gig, he was grateful and relieved because it meant LSU would not sue him for breach of contract and try to recoup lost funding. A few days ago, I received the sad news that a friend of mine had passed away. He was two years younger than me. His passing reminded me of how much he had done for me without ever meaning to.

I owe him a great deal. He took a chance in his own life, opening a wild, unexpected door in mine. I never wrote New Orleans, Louisiana, on a list of places I hoped to live. I had not been planning on this LSU Fellowship my whole life. I thought I would grow old in Puerto Rico. Out of sheer instinct and feeling, I leaped out of my comfort zone and took the unexpected path. I made the most of an opportunity that was not originally intended for me. But I made it mine.

For young doctors and medical students worried they might miss their only chance, I am here to tell you there will be more. You cannot predict or engineer the most important opportunities in your life. They will come. And not always from the places you expect.

There is a time and place for hyperfocus and obsessive planning—those are two things we medical students and doctors do best, after all. But too often, such focus can lead to catastrophizing when things go off the rails. Remember that there is more than one path to success, and when you believe that only one exists, you may miss the existence of the others.

Let my story be a lesson in unexpected opportunities. Be ready for them, embrace them, and make the most of what you have in front of you.

Blazing Your Own Career Path

Throughout this book, you will get a taste of my opinions about what I see as the shortfalls of academic medicine. While I loved working in the hospital setting and learning from more experienced doctors, the competitive attitude and sometimes almost assembly-line style of patient care caused me tremendous stress as a young man.

As I gained confidence in my ability to blaze my trail as a medical practitioner, I opened my private practice—but I did not leave behind all of the education and research aspects of academic medicine when I did so.

I first published this essay in KevinMD in February of 2023 to remind young doctors that their future is in their hands. You are the wielders of medical expertise, and you can craft a career path that contains everything you love about medicine.

You don't have to accept the pre-existing career paths presented to you. And we might find the future of medicine through innovations like this, which prioritize the freedom to practice the humanizing art of medicine alongside research and education.

Combining Academic Medicine and Private Practice: A Success Story

In the United States, physicians are typically categorized as either academics or private practitioners. However, a case can be made that it is possible to construct a career path that incorporates both professional avenues. I was put in an excellent position to realize this during my fellowship at LSU, which structured some parts of its community medicine program in a way that resembled private practice.

I enjoyed my experience as a hospital and clinical fellow. After my fellowship ended, my love affair with academic medicine quickly soured. My director was a rheumatologist, and physical medicine operated under the umbrella of internal medicine at LSU. We were expected to make grand rounds of presentations to some of the world's leading experts. Impressing these experts was the bar for success.

One day, I was assigned to conduct grand rounds by my director. I was still very self-conscious about my accent when speaking English at the time. Moreover, I was actively struggling with panic and anxiety disorders stemming from a major past trauma that I had not yet learned to treat successfully.

The result was that I stood before the prestigious audience at grand rounds with my heart pounding and my voice, legs, and hands shaking. To make things worse, some doctors who had written the textbooks I studied in medical school were in the audience. I felt wildly unprepared to teach them anything new, and afterward, I had the sense that I rushed through my presentation just to be done with it.

Of course, I was magnifying in my mind what had actually taken place.

But, encounters like this can have a powerful effect on a new doctor or professor's self-esteem. I felt I failed my director in one of my most important duties as an assistant professor. Later, the medical school dean found me and congratulated me on doing an "excellent job" on grand rounds. I am unsure if I did better than I thought or if he said this to shore up my confidence.

This anecdote exemplifies the pressure academic medicine can place on doctors. However, there were other conflicts. Additionally, I was not overly fond of the competitive environment of academia, which at times felt like backstabbing. I was aware by this point that competition to publish papers and bring in grant money was so fierce that senior professors often claimed credit for their assistants' work.

New research ideas were commonly kept tightly under wraps for fear of being "scooped" by someone who might procure grant money to fund the research before you did. I saw the pernicious effects of "publish or perish" on full display.

Some people thrive on this type of competition, but none of this suited my personality. So, after a few years as an assistant professor, I moved into private practice.

Private practice, of course, came with its own set of challenges. It was now entirely up to me to bring in my salary, and any lawsuits filed would also be my responsibility rather than falling on the School of Medicine's shoulders. I found myself working more hours with less support. But the pressure to publish and compete with other doctors for publications and grant funding was gone. So I was happy.

Still, I missed a part of academic medicine, and that was teaching students and residents. I had taken pride and pleasure in teaching Fellows the way I had once been taught myself. I decided to do something few other doctors were doing. I created a private practice fellowship program. In this way, I could give opportunities to young doctors, just as a life-changing fellowship opportunity had once been given to me. For a time, my students and I even worked to conduct on-site research and publish articles.

My students saw what it was to work in private practice medicine and learned that it was possible to incorporate some elements of academic medicine while doing so. This was both exciting and fulfilling to me. I had found a best-of-both-worlds scenario.

Some people thrive in the environment of academic medicine. Others are born for private practice. But for those who aren't satisfied, remember that you can blaze your career path as a doctor. It is often possible to build a career path incorporating both aspects.

After all, as a doctor, you are the only genuinely essential requirement for the practice of medicine to happen.

I hope that cultural progress in academic medicine will alleviate some of the burdens of "publish or perish" and create a more supportive, collaborative atmosphere where research can happen with the principal focus on advancing knowledge.

This may be a panacea. But, while the logic of incentivizing research publications and grant funding makes sense, we all know of the problems in academic publishing and grant funding that can sometimes create a divide between the most medically-essential questions and the most well-funded and well-published topics.

The assumption that seminal scientific publications can only be done independently in an academic environment is incorrect. The private practice offers experience, resources, and infrastructure that can enable basic research to be carried out with the proper guardrails and compliance expectations supporting it.

That is a complex and weighty issue for the medical community and colleagues in academic publishing and grant funding to tackle. But for today's physicians and medical students, remember that alternative and innovative paths are always available to you in your career. These hybrid approaches could accelerate the advances in medical research and understanding.

Ultimately, it is up to you to define your career and life direction. What is critical is to understand clearly what is important, relevant, significant, and rewarding to you.

WHEN DEATH COMES FOR THE DOCTOR

In my memoir, *Keep Kicking, Frisco, Keep Kicking*, I discuss the painful death of one of my best friends and role models, Paco. Paco, a fellow physician, always seemed to me to be the ideal doctor and man. He had a beautiful home that he built for his beautiful family. His patients and characters at the local diner loved him and recognized him everywhere he went. He seemed to know how to live with zest and a sense of duty.

Then he got a type of cancer that is almost always rapidly fatal.

News of Paco's diagnosis triggered an internal crisis for me. It underscored the unpredictability of our mortality. If Paco, a man who seemed to be the definition of "doing all the right things," could be cut down in his prime, how could I assume I would live much longer? If he had regrets, which he confided in me despite his exemplary life (one I had long looked toward as a role model for my own), how could I hope to die without regrets?

My essay about why I now imagine my funeral yearly was a runner-up for Doximity's OpMed awards in 2023.

The publication also brought a new insight: some of the physicians who commented became angry with me, with one author even questioning my skill as a doctor for reasons that were logically unclear to me.

I was forced to conclude that facing the specter of mortality is just as difficult for doctors as it is for lay people—perhaps even more so since we have the illusion of power over life and death.

Why This Doctor Imagines His Own Funeral Every Year

I start every year with a practice I learned at a leadership development program. I imagine my own funeral and what my eulogy would be. Sometimes, I even write down the eulogy I would like to have spoken in the event of my death. The key point of the exercise is at the end when you ask yourself if that eulogy would reflect your life.

Leadership coaches recommend this practice because it forces us to ask if we are living the lives we truly want to live. Are we at peace with our choices? What have we neglected in life that we should reconcile while we still have the chance?

Over my career, I have seen three colleagues receive terminal diagnoses. Every time, it should have been a potent reminder that the same could happen to me at any time. Yet I think we, as doctors, often refuse to believe this. Perhaps because we face death so often, we come to believe that we are somehow immortal.

My first experience dealing with death within my professional circle occurred during the second year of residency. Every weekend my attending physician and I got together to play a morning round of tennis doubles with another pair of colleagues. After our match, we always sat by the court's side to chat about our lives.

One Sunday morning, after we finished a very competitive match, one of the other players began to update us on his life. I remember vividly watching this semi-retired pathologist in his late 60s as he casually recounted reading his own tissue sample from a recent colonoscopy.

"I knew right away it wasn't good," he said nonchalantly, staring out over the adjacent tennis courts under the bright blue sky. "Sure enough. Colon cancer. The diagnosis was aggressive and advanced. I'll be dead in three months," he stated almost without emotion.

He died in two.

Several years later, after finishing my fellowship and working on my first job, I reviewed the X-ray films of a patient who was also a fellow physician. The 40-year-old athletic doctor had recently completed an ultramarathon before coming into my colleague's office complaining of back pain.

My colleague's face was grim as he showed me the film for a second opinion. There were several fractures visible on his patient's lumbar and thoracic vertebrae. He knew what that likely meant in an athletic 40-something man, and I confirmed it: It was likely cancer.

I was present when my colleague showed this patient his own X-ray films. As a fellow physician, he knew very well what they meant. Fear and confusion contorted his face. "But how?" he asked. "How could I have cancer?" No one had an answer.

But the most challenging diagnosis for me to witness was that of my best friend. A fellow physician in his late 30s, he was one of the most driven people I had ever known. He had created his well-respected medical practice and provided a good life for his beautiful young family. While I struggled with unhealthy habits and sweated over work-life balance, he was one of those people who seemed to do everything right.

One late summer Sunday afternoon, he called to tell me he was seeing a chiropractor because of severe low back pain. Then he stopped picking up the phone for weeks.

When he finally called back, he was crying. He had learned weeks ago that he had been diagnosed with pancreatic cancer, which had already metastasized throughout his body. He was only now coming to terms with the diagnosis.

He was a different man the first time he agreed to see me after his diagnosis. He looked defeated and sad. He was quiet and withdrawn. The cheerful, vivacious man I knew was gone.

I took him to run some errands. During that brief trip, I asked him how he felt. He confessed to me he felt afraid and angry. He regretted having put all his efforts into building a successful medical practice at the expense of family time. Last summer, he skipped an overseas trip with his wife and children to attend to business needs.

I asked him what treatments his care team was trying. "You know as well as I do that I'm dying," he said. "There's no cure for this type of cancer. I'm not going to see my children grow up." All his life, this friend had been a health fanatic. He was fastidious about what he ate. The few unkind words he spoke were usually directed at people who didn't care for their bodies. The irony was painful and cruel. It made me cold with the implications.

We may wonder about each of these doctors' journeys to confronting their own mortality. Was the first man so at peace with his life that he accepted death readily, or was he deep in denial? Had the athletic doctor ever considered the possibility that death could come for him soon? Would my best friend have made different choices the previous summer if he had known what was in store for him the next year?

Steve Jobs once said, "Remembering that I'll be dead soon is the most important tool I've ever encountered to help me make the big choices in life. Because almost everything — all external expectations, all pride, all fear of embarrassment or failure — these things just fall away in the face of death, leaving only what is truly important. Remembering that you will die is the best way to avoid the trap of thinking you have something to lose. You are already naked."

How can we treat the remembrance of our own mortality as something liberating that frees us to focus on what is truly important?

The prospect of death will likely never be pleasant, but by confronting it head-on before it confronts us, we may stop it from catching us unprepared. We will not fear death when our focus is on a life well-lived.

What do you hope is said at your funeral? Are you living the life you want?

WHEN IT ACTUALLY IS A ZEBRA

In medical school, a common adage is, "When you hear hoofbeats, think of horses, not zebras." That translates to, "Don't assume a patient has a rare condition when a common one would adequately explain their symptoms."

This is generally a good adage for doctors and patients trying to diagnose themselves. Hear this, WebMD fans: if your newly developed symptoms could be adequately explained by cancer *or* stomach flu, it is overwhelmingly likely that it's the flu.

But as doctors, we sometimes see patients for whom the first-line treatments don't work. What do we do when a patient has a condition with no generally accepted treatment? What about when generally accepted treatments are not providing enough relief? Rare diseases do walk among us, and it may sometimes be within our scope of duty to recommend our patients to less well-studied or widely accepted treatment modalities to do all we can for them.

In the case of the patient I discuss in my following essay, at the time I treated her, the treatment called prolotherapy had a relatively poor reputation in the medical community. There was so little empirical support for its use that some went so far as to call it pseudoscience. But it was the best I could offer this patient after first-line approaches had failed. When practicing the human art of medicine, thinking and acting in unconventional ways is sometimes necessary to fulfill our duty to our patients.

In the years since, additional studies about its effectiveness have come out, to the point that the Mayo Clinic has tentatively endorsed prolotherapy. My reflection on prescribing this treatment to a patient with Ehlers-Danlos Syndrome before it was a widely accepted treatment course first appeared in KevinMD in May 2023.

Finding Hope and Relief: A Physical Therapist's Journey with Chronic Pain and Ehlers-Danlos Syndrome (EDS)

The day Ann entered my clinic, I had already been practicing pain management for over ten years. A 40-something physical therapist, she had a warm smile, a positive attitude—and chronic pain in every part of her back.

Twenty-five years earlier, Ann had been inspired to go into physical therapy to help her family members who suffered from severe chronic pain to the point of disability. However, to her dismay, upon graduating from her PT program, she found that her physical therapy training did little to help herself, as she began to suffer from pronounced chronic pain in her early 20s. The usual methods for treating musculoskeletal injuries were not getting the job done.

In her late 20s, Ann was finally diagnosed with Ehlers-Danlos Syndrome (EDS). In this often underdiagnosed condition, the body's collagen is fragile. The most common symptoms leading to a diagnosis are musculoskeletal pain and joint hypermobility, although many subtypes of the condition exist depending on the type of collagen affected. EDS patients may also present with unexplained bruising, cardiac valve problems, ruptured arteries and organs, hip dislocation, kyphoscoliosis, muscle hypotonicity, eye and tooth problems, and more.

Many patients with EDS struggle to get diagnosed. Physicians may assume that patients with hypermobility cannot truly experience meaningful joint and muscle pain since conventional musculoskeletal problems often come with a restricted range of motion. Some may attribute spontaneous joint dislocations to athletic activities or be unaware of the other symptoms that EDS can cause.

Once diagnosed, the result is a mixed bag of good and bad news. As Ann had observed, physical therapy may not completely resolve EDS symptoms. Her primary care doctor thought it had failed to relieve pain. Ann faced an increased risk of pain from her EDS.

Fortunately for me, I knew a doctor who could help. My colleague, Dr. Felix Linetsky, had successfully treated several EDS and joint hypermobility patients with RIT.

RIT, short for "regenerative injection therapy," a term coined by Dr. Linetsky in 1991, is also sometimes called prolotherapy or sclerotherapy. The procedure involves injecting chemical or biological agents into connective tissues suffering from injury or chronic pain that is not resolved with other treatments. The injections are intended to stimulate the patient's body to heal the injury in the same way that using adjuvants in vaccines strengthens the immune response to a pathogen.

Some practitioners have taken this one step further by including stem cells, platelet-rich plasma, or fat tissue from the patient's own body in RIT injections, hoping these biological components will lend an extra helping hand to healing factors and regenerative tissue.

Although the practice of injecting connective tissue to stimulate healing has existed for over a century, RIT or prolotherapy has a new body of evidence regarding its effectiveness. While some studies suggesting its effectiveness have been criticized for flawed methodology, more recent well-designed studies have shown evidence for its effectiveness in treating low back pain, lateral epicondylitis, and Achilles tendonitis.

Many doctors are aware that some proponents have overstated RIT's benefits and are unaware of studies that have appeared since 2015, suggesting benefits for several forms of musculoskeletal pain that do not respond sufficiently to first-line treatments.

Unfortunately, the use of RIT in Ehlers-Danlos Syndrome has not been rigorously studied. This is a byproduct of an overall lack of attention to EDS, a condition that can be difficult to diagnose and meaningfully treat by the medical establishment.

The use of RIT has not been studied in EDS but has been studied in hypermobility joint syndrome. Like HDS, hypermobility joint syndrome does not have specific genetic markers; some authors consider them the same entity with a strong genetic component.

When the underlying problem is fragile collagen that may not respond well to traditional exercise or physical therapy methods, it can be easy for doctors to feel helpless and not want to think too hard about the patients they feel unable to help.

However, Dr. Linetsky and I believe it is precisely these patients for whom we must explore all potential avenues of treatment.

We have seen more than a few patients in our practices who have expressed profound relief for their challenging conditions with RIT and expressed frustration that conventional doctors often dismiss or even condemn these treatments. Well-known medical institutions like the Mayo Clinic offer RIT as platelet-rich plasma (PRP), bone marrow aspirate (BMAC), and other methods.

When we already know that symptoms are severe and are not responding to first-line treatments, safe treatment may warrant exploration, even if it is not mainstream or widely accepted.

After seeing Dr. Linetsky, Ann began to report improvements in her pain, mobility, and ability to lead an everyday life. She continues to see him well into her 60s.

Having an accurate impact assessment of Ann's condition and improvement based on the RIT treatments is challenging. There are no large and rigorously controlled clinical studies on the effect of RIT treatment on EDS.

Therefore, such clinical studies must be supported to precisely determine this promising approach's potential for this type of patient. The welfare of our patients greatly depends on the physician's ability and willingness to consider diagnoses and treatments beyond what may be seemingly evident from initial observation.

Names and details have been changed to protect the patient's privacy.

When Surgery Isn't Necessary

As someone who considers himself to be a health and fitness educator, my ego was a little bruised when I injured myself while exercising at home during the COVID-19 pandemic. My ego was not the only damage: the damage to my knee, in the words of a surgeon who reviewed my MRI, was quite impressive.

If not for the pandemic, my surgery might have been scheduled immediately. But with elective surgeries on indefinite pause as an infection control measure, I had the opportunity to try something else. I set out to rehab my knee to normal levels of function without surgical intervention.

The conventional wisdom among many doctors was that this was a crazy undertaking. The physical damage to my knee was so profound that, in their opinion, it should not have been possible for it to function normally without surgical repair to fix the mechanical tears and damage.

But I came from another perspective: as a long-time physiatrist involved with rehab, I knew that a patient's adherence to their rehab routine was often a *more* important determiner of recovery than the surgeon's report.

It is easy to see why the medical community might be more comfortable focusing on surgery than rehab for patients. After all, rehab compliance largely depends on the patient's own choices, and managing patients' behavior at home can range from time-intensive to impossible. But for patients who are dedicated to their recovery, rehab represents a vastly underappreciated well of potential for regaining mobility and function, with or without surgery.

My reflection on the power of rehabilitation exercise first appeared in KevinMD in July of 2023.

Optimize Your Knee Injury Recovery Without Surgery

Recently, growing attention has been given to the fact that some types of surgery may be overrated. This article, citing dozens of studies showing that some orthopedic surgeries popular in past decades had no better results than non-invasive treatments.[1]

This issue is deeply personal to me. In 2020, during the pandemic, I sustained an injury to my left knee, experiencing severe pain, swelling, and loss of motion. An MRI revealed a posterior cruciate ligament (PCL) avulsion fraction of the tibial plateau with a small fragment, a posterior horn medial meniscus tear, and strains to both the anterior and posterior cruciate ligaments (ACL and PCL) with a partial tear to the plantar and popliteus muscles.

---

1. Hargrove, T. (2022, March 5). *Many orthopedic surgeries don't work*. Physio Network. https://physio-network.com/blog/many-orthopedic-surgeries-dont-work/

An initial evaluation by an orthopedic surgeon determined that surgery was necessary to restore normal function to my knee and resume my regular physical activities, such as long-distance running. However, as a physiatrist, I believed conservative treatment could be effective. Additionally, the uncertainties surrounding hospitalization and surgery during the pandemic played a role in my decision.

Fortunately, I had been involved in studying the building and rebuilding of the body from two angles: that of physiatry and that of bodybuilding. Utilizing this knowledge, I created an exercise program to regain full range of motion and weight-bearing in my injured knee. In the summer of 2022, I successfully ran a high-altitude marathon in Machu Picchu without any complications or restrictions.

The treatment of intra-articular ligament tears requires careful evaluation to determine the best approach. Some cases may indeed require surgery. Neglecting surgery in such instances may lead to long-term consequences, including a higher risk of re-injury and chronic instability. Seeking medical advice and considering all options is crucial before deciding on the most suitable course of action.

Non-surgical treatments have been challenging to study due to their complexity and the time required for completion. More high-quality research is needed to compare these treatments to surgical outcomes for injuries similar to mine.

For other injury types, research has indicated a higher risk and lower reward profile for surgery. Therefore, non-surgical interventions should receive more attention if my injury can recover without surgery, and if certain surgeries have been overestimated in their effectiveness.

One area that researchers should explore is the impact of anti-inflammatory diets and lifestyle changes on injury recovery. Personally, I firmly believe in research demonstrating how certain foods can increase or decrease inflammatory markers. During my knee injury and recovery, I took supplements like high-EPA and -DHA fish oil, turmeric, and vitamin D3 with K2. Notably, I did not immediately connect this to my successful healing process.

However, later on, I learned that my son, when seeking treatment for his back pain at a regenerative medicine clinic, was advised to follow an anti-inflammatory diet and supplement regimen for weeks before his visit. They made it clear that they would not proceed with treatment if he did not follow this protocol, as inflammation was deemed a leading cause of treatment failure in their back pain patients. His treatment was effective and relieved his persistent back pain.

On the surface, this approach makes common sense. A growing body of evidence demonstrates that certain foods, which have become increasingly prevalent in American diets in recent decades, contribute to systemic inflammation. We are discovering more mechanisms for this, such as the creation of Specialized Pro-resolving Mediators (SPMs) in response to consuming certain omega-3 fatty acids, and the possibility of an autoimmune response to Neu5G incorporated into our cells due to the consumption of red meat.

As health care providers, our primary goal is to facilitate the healing process for our patients. We employ various treatments, including medications and interventions, to create the optimal environment for recovery. However, when it comes to rehabilitating injuries, we often neglect to consider the impact of diet, despite the well-known adage "you are what you eat."

It is crucial to recognize that the raw materials for growth and healing in our bodies are derived from the foods we consume. As such, we should place emphasis on understanding our patients' dietary habits and advising them accordingly. Currently, we tend to address specific dietary regimens only when treating obesity or gastric distress, but we should extend this approach to all patients to promote optimal health and healing.

Have we given up on advising patients on diet because many of them must follow basic recommendations about consuming enough fruits and vegetables? This would be a mistake. Providing specific advice tailored to a particular upcoming medical event may be perceived differently than general advice that everyone should always follow.

Or have we, as medical professionals, neglected the role of nutrition because much of what we are learning about the role of different foods in healing and disease processes is new? The era of molecular medicine has led to the discovery of hundreds, if not thousands, of new biochemical pathways, shedding light on the sometimes-confusing results of diet studies from the last century. However, many of these discoveries have yet to be put into widespread practice in clinical or dietary guidelines.

By shifting back to personalized exercise and dietary regimens for patients facing acute illness and injury, we may observe superior risk-reward profiles compared to what we currently see with surgical interventions alone. Moreover, surgical interventions, with their long list of potential risks and side effects, may prove to be less common than we previously assumed.

In conclusion, the decision to pursue surgical or non-surgical treatment for knee ligament tears should be based on individual circumstances and after consultation with a health care provider. This is precisely why it is incumbent upon us as providers to consider all possible interventions and all available medical knowledge when presenting our patients with their treatment options.

When we recognize that surgery alone has often historically proven to be less than optimal, it becomes essential to investigate all the new science available to us, including increasingly nuanced findings about the effects of food and exercise on our healing processes.

WHEN RESPECT BECOMES A CHALLENGE

In recent years, medicine has become an increasingly high-stress, high-pressure field. When the stakes of an error can be life or death and doctors face mounting pressures from external forces, it can be easy to snap.

Yet in medicine, more than in many other fields, respect for patients and colleagues is essential. We cannot obtain favorable outcomes if we do not respect the human person.

It is incumbent on each of us to become a locus of control—a place where a culture of respect is born and disrespect stops.

In August 2023, KevinMD published this essay in which I recount seeing a surgeon lose his temper during surgery after a piece of essential equipment malfunctioned. I meditate on how, despite mounting pressures on medical practitioners, respect for patients is essential—even, and perhaps especially, when the patient is believed to be unconscious and unable to defend themselves.

Patient Respect in Medicine: Ensuring Well-Being and Trust

Treating patients with respect and dignity is essential to the medical profession. This is true even when the patient lies unconscious in the operating room. It seems unnecessary to stress the importance of creating a secure and comfortable environment to ease the patient's anxiety and stress and develop confidence.

Respect is also crucial to promote successful outcomes. By prioritizing these values, medical professionals can ensure that patients feel valued and cared for, even in the most vulnerable situations.

Every medical care step needs respect for the patient and their welfare. This can be seen in an operating room's spoken and unspoken expectations. Operating room culture emphasizes precision, efficiency, and teamwork, with each team member playing a crucial role in ensuring the procedure's success.

Effective communication is critical; everyone must collaborate seamlessly to provide patients with the best care. Every precaution is taken to keep the environment clean and safe. Overall, the operating room culture demands the highest professionalism and dedication from everyone involved.

I remember being a second-year physical medicine and rehabilitation resident at the VA medical center, where I witnessed the negative impact of an operating room's dysfunctional culture. During one of my first orthopedic surgeries as a resident, the leading surgeon encountered a problem with the drill used for a total hip replacement.

Although the drill was still operational, it malfunctioned and caused frustration for the attending physician. He shared his concern with the chief operating room nurse, who suggested writing a work order but added that the drill could not be replaced if it still was functioning.

The attending physician was increasingly frustrated as this was not the first time a surgical tool malfunctioned. Despite receiving the same response repeatedly, he resorted to hitting the drill with a metal hammer. The surgeon was yelling and using profanity, and neglecting the patient's welfare. He derisively asserted that the drill was unusable now and demanded a replacement.

The nurse was taken aback and irate. She warned him that she would submit a formal grievance to the Chief of Staff. The behavior mentioned above may have resulted in an extension of the elective surgery, ultimately leading to potential complications.

This anecdote is in no way typical. However, the situation exemplifies the loss in patient perspective that could lead to unsafe environments for patients and health care professionals. A lack of communication, respect, and accountability can result in mistakes and patient harm.

Hospitals and surgical teams must strive for a positive and functional culture in the operating room, with the ultimate focus on the safety and well-being of patients. This requires a cohesive and effective team effort.

During my extensive training to become an interventional physiatrist, I observed disrespectful attitudes and conduct while performing outpatient procedures at the surgical center. I witnessed one of the medical professionals present during the procedure behaving in a derogatory manner toward patients. This included making fun of tattooed patients or commenting on their appearance. Often criticizing poor hygiene and foul odors.

This behavior can upset patients and worsen their health care system experience. All professionals need to treat their patients with respect and dignity, regardless of their personal beliefs. It was disappointing and concerning to see that some individuals needed to uphold the crucial standards of maintaining a professional and respectful demeanor, despite the significance of doing so.

As medical professionals, we must prioritize the well-being and comfort of our patients, and disrespectful behavior has no place in our field.

In recent years, many doctors have that disrespectful behavior in medical settings may threaten patient safety. Some of this rise has been.[1] Reports of pressures from administrative bodies who often have conflicting interests have been discussed among doctors for .[2] If this is true, it's profoundly concerning news.

---

1. *Disrespectful behaviors in healthcare have increased during pandemic.* ECRI. (n.d.). https://www.ecri.org/press/disrespectful-behaviors-in-healthcare-have-increased-during-pandemic

2. Chen, P. W. (2010, April 29). *Fueling the anger of doctors.* The New York Times. https://www.nytimes.com/2010/04/30/health/29chen.html

There's no end to the tug-of-war between financially motivated health care systems, financially motivated insurance companies, and patient welfare, which often sees doctors scrutinized and berated from three directions simultaneously.

The need for professionalism and team cohesiveness applies when speaking to patients and when the patient is unaware of the surroundings.

The manner of behavior around a sedated patient matters, though they may not know how they are treated. The commentaries, atmosphere, and music can impact the patient's well-being. I will admit that there is room to relax and seek relief from stressful situations. But when that informality comes at the expense of the patient, particularly in a disrespectful manner, it does something long-term to the medical provider that carries even to other patients.

The experiences I have shared are a few examples of the importance of the relationship between doctor and patient, even when that patient is sedated. The consistency of attitude under all circumstances and in all medical environments ensures the resiliency and genuineness of character that our patients can feel. This is of great value and worth the effort to develop, maintain, and protect.

The topic of doctors and nurses engaging in seemingly disrespectful behavior when they think patients are not looking has been raised frequently. The "black humor" of the medical profession, which occurs when doctors and nurses joke about devastating diseases to cope with the trauma they witness daily, has become infamous. Some have pointed out that this coping mechanism is necessary for people whose full-time job deals with the worst-case scenarios that most people only have to witness a few times.

But the cases I cite are examples of the exquisite care we must take as health care workers not to allow our coping mechanisms to affect our patients. We must treat our patients how we want our loved ones to be treated in life and death.

CREATING A LEGACY: SELFISH OR SELFLESS?

In August 2023, Doximity OpMed published this essay about my grandfather's legacy and my own. In the essay, I discuss seeking public recognition for my grandfather, who made a foundational difference in medicine in Puerto Rico, and about creating a legacy for myself by which I may be remembered.

The most exciting part of this essay was the responses it created. Many healthcare providers commented, suggesting that it was selfish to want to do things that would be remembered and that a doctor's job is simply to treat patients every day.

While I agree that treating patients in the clinic daily is a worthwhile way to spend one's life, I also challenge the assumption that this practice alone is enough. After all, having a legacy is to have created significant change. To be remembered means to have changed the lives of many people in some significant way.

At the same time, we must be mindful of the harm that can be caused by unscrupulously seeking credit or attention for ourselves. History is full of examples of lives lost and atrocities committed because unscrupulous doctors wished to have their names attached to a discovery, even if it meant delaying progress on lifesaving cures or conducting research on patients without their consent.

Should we, then, seek to build legacies for ourselves? Will thinking about how to do so drive us to do bigger, bolder, and better things to leave the world better than we found it? Or will it lead to vainglorious exercises in which our public image becomes more important to us than the real-world effects of our actions?

I will leave it to you, dear reader, to read and decide.

What Does it Mean to Have a Legacy As a Doctor?

At the core of it, all doctors are healers. Some of us practice as clinicians, touching and treating individual patients day in and day out. Some of us teach the future of our profession, and even more of us still conduct important scientific research in laboratories and other settings.

Medicine has always been more of a vocation than a career. It attracts purpose-driven people. Whether or not it always feels this way — we all became physicians because we thought this path would allow us to help others.

One of my first mentors was an academic. He was the medical school's dean at Louisiana State University, giving me my first job in the U.S. One day, I caught a peek at his CV. It was hundreds of pages long. I asked this doctor why he would have created a document like this one. I thought he was going on the teaching market elsewhere. However, his answer surprised me. He told me he wanted to be remembered once his time ended.

Recently, I was able to create a Wikipedia page for my undefined.undefined But this turned out to be more challenging than straightforward. It was a struggle to convince Wikipedia editors that his impact was significant enough to have his own page, even though he was a renowned author of both scientific articles and poems, served as dean of the only school of pharmacy on the island of Puerto Rico for more than 40 years, and founded a museum bearing his name.

In the end, I could do it, and now there is a page highlighting my grandfather's life accomplishments on Wikipedia.

The conscious legacy building may seem like a narcissistic endeavor, divorced from the altruism that characterizes many doctors and their work. My thesis is that we are doing a disservice (maybe large, maybe small) to ourselves and our patients if we continue thinking about what we leave behind.

Unlike my grandfather, I don't teach or do research. I see patients. Each is their own world to explore and their own opportunity to make a difference. I take great pains to hear them out, explore the proper treatment, and follow through on care. I should be satisfied to leave it at that. After all, what is more rewarding than changing a single patient's life for the better? I certainly get immense joy from it.

This got me thinking about the question of legacy.

Not long ago, some of my fellow doctors suggested that it was unrealistic to have a goal to make a difference that is remembered after one's life is over. Nevertheless, I disagree. What does it mean to have a legacy? It means you have changed something that persists after you die.

My experience documenting and publicizing my grandfather's legacy makes it apparent why many people feel that leaving a legacy is unrealistic. The fact remains that even if one accomplishes a great deal in life, it's hard to fathom how you will be remembered for it. This begs the question: What was my grandfather's true legacy — the many lasting and significant contributions he made to Puerto Rican society and the medical world in general, or the record of a Wikipedia page commemorating those facts?

Many of us in the medical community are motivated to study medicine to help people. Some of us are motivated for other reasons, then feel a sense of responsibility once given the tools to practice medicine and contribute to medical science.

Either way, we have choices. Two of them are that 1) we can take action to try to alleviate suffering where we see it, fix systemic problems when we find them, and contribute to the world's medical knowledge where we see knowledge gaps, or 2) we can decide that it's enough just to get by and do a good job that is satisfying and productive.

Legacies are not necessarily achieved by making the best grades or publishing the most papers but by doing what others neglect. They are made by doing or studying what has been dismissed as impossible, undetected, or unimportant. They are made by going against the current, often in the face of criticism.

In part, because I grew up under my grandfather's influence, who was famous in my homeland long before he existed on Wikipedia, the question of legacy has always been acute. How could I possibly live up to my grandfather's legacy?

By making tough decisions to impact those around me positively, I have stumbled into what I can recognize as the beginnings of a legacy. I have created a "hybrid" career path allowing physicians like myself to access the benefits of academic and private practice endeavors.

In recent years, I have become an author and speaker on the human side of medicine. I have the established orthodoxy of a professional setting for academic research. Still, I have contributed to how the medical community thinks and feels about the experiences of doctors and patients — a vital and fraught topic in the American medical system of today.

This is not to impress but to highlight the potential that everyone has to leave a legacy. No matter how limited you feel in your opportunities or responsibilities, there are ways to make a difference. Fixing the problems you feel compelled to lies in first identifying them.

So the pertinent questions are: What difference can you make in this world before you leave it? How many people will say that you are crazy for even trying? What do you have to gain from listening to them?

Legacies happen not merely because of ability or hard work but because we combine those with a sense of purpose. This is fortunate for us, as having a sense of purpose is also a significant correlate of good mental health and life satisfaction. We can expect to reap personal rewards for acting in ways that change the world even if no one remembers that we did it.

Mark Twain summed it well: "The two most important days in your life are the day you were born and the day you find out why."

WHAT KIDS CAN TEACH DOCTORS

As so many parents so often report, having children changed me. But not in the ways I expected; I gained a whole new understanding of love. But I also learned things I never expected from watching my children as they learned to be human beings.

Pediatrics is a famously tricky discipline, partly because pediatric patients often lack the communication skills we expect of adults. Diagnoses must often be made based on the children's body language and facial expressions, and pediatric patients must be prompted with careful patience to tell us where it hurts. We must be exquisitely gentle with them, for they frighten easily.

Yet isn't that true, to some extent, of all patients with whom we are in a doctor-patient relationship? Shouldn't we exercise the same kind of sensitivity and patience toward anyone who comes to us seeking care? It may be a challenging thing to do. But if parents can do it every day, why can't we?

My reflections on what my children taught me about practicing medicine appeared in Doximity's OpMed column in August of 2023.

What My Children Have Taught Me About Medicine

Throughout my professional journey, I've received guidance from prominent figures in the personal success industry, including Anthony Robbins, Deepak Chopra, and Robin Sharma. While I have learned much from these experts, their lessons pale compared to those from my kids.

Having children changes a person's perspective on life irrevocably. We get to experience vicariously what it is like to know the world for the first time. We develop a profound sense of responsibility for the welfare and importance of these tiny humans that can translate into how we view other individuals. No one is as important to you as your kids, and it can be challenging to comprehend how vital anyone is until you've known the feeling of having children.

Having children requires a person to learn specific communication skills. Children cannot articulate their symptoms to you for the first few years of their lives.

You must learn to read their body language and responses to determine where it hurts and what emotions they are experiencing. Such skills can be invaluable in the clinic, where many patients struggle to articulate or are unwilling to share such details with their doctor. I was amazed to see the previously mystifying behavior of certain patients become decipherable after spending a few years shepherding a toddler through unspoken hunger and tummy aches.

Learning to communicate as a parent improved my communication skills with my patients immensely. With children, there is no reasonable expectation that they know what to expect of you or that they should clearly articulate their feelings without being prompted.

A skill develops, then, in gently handling another human being, warning them, obtaining their consent, and listening to their concerns. While it might be ideal and possible for some people to develop these skills outside of parenthood, for most of us, parenthood is the first time in our lives that that much patience and sensitivity is required.

Parenthood is a 24/7 crash course in the attitude and skills that a perfect society would teach us all as young adults but that our current society unfortunately does not.

In addition, my children have changed the way I see and treat myself.

When we receive medical training in med school, we are not taught to value self-care.

While the system has improved since some of us older doctors were in training, many still argue that the "resiliency modules" mandated by many medical schools today do not meaningfully improve self-care, as adding more items to a medical student's to-do list is unlikely to result in an actual, meaningful increase in healthy eating, sleeping, or exercise.

Having children is another story. When I had a cardiac scare in my 40s, front and center in my mind was this: Would I be there to see my children finish growing up? What would they do without me? I could not abandon them. And so, I could not die.

The same responsibility must apply, in a less intense way, to our patients. We cannot serve our patients optimally or care for them if we are ill, chronically sleep-deprived, or deceased. We must take the maintenance of our bodies as the vehicles of our lives quite seriously, with a deliberateness about the daily hands-on practicalities that few young doctors display.

Whatever we may be taught in medical school about having to perform an impossible number of tasks to be good doctors, we certainly cannot be good doctors if we're *dead*.

On top of this, children and patients can both motivate us in another way. Children and adults alike learn from our examples, not our lectures. They are far more likely to do as we *do* than as we *tell* them to do. For this reason, self-care becomes necessary to ensure that our children, or our patients, practice good self-care of their own. Lecturing them about eating healthy while surviving on coffee and donuts does not work.

As a healthcare professional, I understand the fear and uncertainty of medical decisions, especially when it involves one's children. I remember signing a consent form for my youngest child's outpatient surgery and feeling overwhelmed by all the potential risks. It made me realize the importance of discussing any medical procedure thoroughly with my patients and addressing any concerns.

I also take it upon myself to remember that every patient is someone's child.

It is fair to say that you care about your children's health in a way you are unlikely to care about strangers automatically. When you are accustomed to caring for a tiny human who is deeply important to you, the way you relate to those who are hurting or sick in general changes. For me, it is impossible to see a patient merely as an adult stranger; they are also someone's child.

I must credit my children for helping me become a better doctor in all these ways. I have found that the incentive to develop emotional intelligence, sensitivity, and vigilance for caring for strangers was different after experiencing the daily life of a parent.

In sum, the heightened sense of empathy and the experience guiding young humans through their first experiences of life is invaluable to my medical practice. It has had a profound effect on my journey, leading me to delve into holistic health, regenerative medicine, and other healing modalities that were not, strictly speaking, on my med-school syllabus.

As my children have grown, they have taught me in new ways. Witnessing their journeys of struggle and triumph throughout their teen and adult years has given me a renewed appreciation for life and the power of the human spirit. I have broadened my horizons as a parent in ways I would never have if confined by my narrow views and expectations of life.

My children have been my most excellent teachers, and I will be forever grateful to them for allowing me to accompany them on their journeys through life.

Are We Rational In Our Use of Psychiatric Assessments?

In 2023, I was approached by a medical student concerned about the system used by local hospitals to decide whether to authorize patients for surgery. The algorithm required that patients show specific results on psychiatric assessments to be approved for surgery—but my student feared that this system was ruling out patients who needed treatment. I shared his concerns based on my own experiences of patients being denied treatment.

In September 2023, KevinMD published my essay on this matter, in which I questioned whether psychiatric assessments were being used wisely or discriminatorily. I also did my best to remind the audience that questioning the value of our tools and whether they are being used in a way that obtains the best results is the only way things get better in medicine.

Debating the Role of Psychiatric Assessments in Medical Decisions

I recently had an incident involving a long-time patient. This particular encounter proved to be challenging. The patient had chronic pain for years and had already exhausted all conventional treatment options. Ironically, he was otherwise healthy and fit. His recalcitrant condition made him a prime candidate to be treated with a spinal cord stimulator (SCS).

An SCS is an implantable device with two electrode leads connected to a battery-powered pulse generator. The electrodes are inserted into the epidural space and positioned alongside the ascending pain fibers at the level of the nerve causing symptoms. The generator sends pulses to stimulate the nerve and block pain signals from reaching the brain. SCSs are ideal for treating neuropathic pain,

Complex regional pain syndrome, and failed back surgery syndrome. SCSs are an excellent treatment option, particularly in cases where other approaches have proven unsuccessful. However, the treatment is not without risks and associated costs.

There was just one problem. The standard requirement is to complete a psychiatric evaluation to get approval for the surgery. Furthermore, as it turned out, doing so was against this patient's religious beliefs.

My patient was a member of one of several religious organizations that consider the entire practice of psychiatry forbidden. In some cases, such patients believe that interacting with the mental health system in any way will jeopardize their spiritual or physical well-being by showing a lack of faith in their God. He apologetically informed me that if taking a psychiatric evaluation was the only way for him to get a spinal cord stimulator, he'd have to do without one.

Although somewhat taken aback by his treatment refusal, I could empathize with his dilemma. This also made me reflect on the purpose of these psychiatric evaluations. Since mental illnesses often manifest as physical pain, the spinal stimulator screening protocol addressed potential psychiatric causes of pain before considering a potentially dangerous and costly surgery.

However, if this is true, why were psychiatric evaluations not required for other medical interventions routinely used to treat chronic pain in patients? What was unique about this particular procedure? Since psychiatric comorbidities can worsen almost every known medical symptom, shouldn't we have been screening patients for psychiatric issues before any non-emergency surgery if our concern was ensuring patients received the least invasive treatments possible?

The implications were troubling. Was the requirement for the psychiatric evaluation related to the still-widespread perception that many chronic pain sufferers are "crazy" or "faking"? I thought back to a documentary I'd recently watched.

Take Care of Maya is a documentary about a young girl suffering from complex regional pain syndrome who was accused by medical staff of faking her pain. Those who took an oath to treat her pain dismissed her as hysterical even as they billed her insurance for the same diagnosis they told her she concocted in her head.

Too many medical providers still believe that chronic pain with no apparent mechanical source cannot be genuine. Was this why we were compelled to check our patients for psychiatric diagnoses before performing this surgery?

Another possible reason for this screening requirement lies in the for-profit insurance industry. It is widely known that insurers often invest considerable effort to identify reasons to deny coverage for treatments. Psychiatric evaluations provide a convenient tool for this. Insurance companies have implemented psychiatric evaluation requirements for numerous surgeries, including organ transplants, bariatric surgery, in vitro fertilization, and cosmetic surgery.

In some cases, the rationale was that behavioral changes are needed after surgery to ensure good outcomes. Some have argued that patients seeking cosmetic and other elective surgeries should undergo a mental health exam before going under the knife, as they need to be "protected from" their own choices.

Others have argued that, since donor organs should go to patients with the best chance of surviving transplantation, evaluating a patient's psychiatric prognosis before giving an organ to them instead of another patient is warranted.

I agree that psychiatric assessments are warranted under certain conditions and can play a role in preventing unnecessary risk-prone procedures. Nevertheless, the extent of implementation with such a broad spectrum of applications begins to sound overly Draconian.

Eligibility for appropriate and best medical care should not depend on subjective assessments that may be biased toward denying care for non-medical reasons. A key question is: What standards are used to judge the correlation between psychiatric distress and surgical outcomes?

A literature review titled "Psychiatric Screening for Spinal Cord Stimulation for Complex Regional Pain Syndrome" documents 15 psychological screening tools studied. This review showed inconclusive evidence linking screening test scores with predicting SCS outcomes. This means there is no apparent benefit to requiring a psychiatric evaluation to qualify for this procedure in practice.

Psychiatric evaluations could be a legitimate and valuable tool for treating the whole patient. That becomes especially true with a robust, evidence-based system for providing psychiatrically distressed patients with mental health treatment and community support. Unfortunately, that is not in place in the United States today. So, we must be exceedingly careful in deciding who determines who is "eligible" for treatment and what criteria we use to make that decision.

I advocate for further clarity and standards on who decides whether a patient must undergo a psychiatric evaluation. These fundamental decisions for critical health care should be detached from any conflict of interest that may arise from financial considerations.

What if research reveals that these evaluations are causing harm by denying treatment to patients who would still benefit from the surgery despite their psychological difficulties? What do we do with cases like my patient, who refuses to receive a psychiatric evaluation due to religious convictions before the procedure?

At the very least, we should demand scientifically sound evidence that denying patients treatment due to their mental state is in the best interest of the patient. We must be mindful of who decides who receives treatment and who doesn't. We must be careful not to do harm because of the stigma around mental health.

Is Ozempic All It's Cracked Up to Be?

In 2023, I published a new edition of my book, "Drop the Fat Diet: 12 Steps to a Leaner You Forever." KevinMD published an excerpt from this book on the newly popular drug semaglutide, often known by its brand name, Ozempic.

As a doctor who speaks frequently about the importance of fitness to health, many people have expected that I would be ecstatic about the weight loss effects of Ozempic, which mimics the "satiety hormone" glucagon. However, I am concerned. While Ozempic may curb overeating and lead to weight loss, it does nothing to improve nutrition or access to healthy food. And weight loss, as I so often argue in my "Drop the Fat Diet" books, is not the same as health or fitness.

Ozempic: Miracle Drug or a Band-Aid for Obesity?

Semaglutide, a medication often marketed as Ozempic, Wegovy, or Rybelsus, has gained immense popularity in recent years. This is especially true in an age where diabetes and obesity are on the rise. The medication is being seen as a panacea for effortless weight loss. Some doctors and activists have hailed it as a miracle drug that can help shift the conversation around obesity from a judgmental approach to a disease model of metabolic illness.

Obesity, a condition characterized by excessive body fat, is a complex and multifactorial issue that has become a public health concern worldwide. Several factors, including genetics, hormones, stress, and food availability, influence the development of obesity. The interplay between these factors can lead to an imbalance in energy intake and expenditure, resulting in an accumulation of body fat.

While genetic and hormonal factors may predispose individuals to obesity, environmental factors such as food availability and stress can exacerbate the condition. Therefore, a comprehensive approach that addresses individual and environmental factors is necessary to prevent and manage obesity. There is often a tendency to treat obese patients judgmentally.

One reason behind this is that obesity is now associated with poverty. People who can only afford processed foods, work too much to cook but do not earn enough to buy expensive pre-made healthy meals, or who have high stress levels due to living in poverty are much more likely to be obese than the wealthy and privileged individuals who we see being celebrated for their fitness and beauty in magazines.

Many celebrity influencers have faced public backlash for promoting their "diet and fitness secrets" while taking all the credit for themselves as experts, even though they are supported by a team of nutritionists, chefs, and personal trainers.

Several healthy meal delivery services claim to be affordable, but in reality, they charge more than $10 per meal per person, which can add up to over $200 per week for one person to eat three meals per day, seven days per week. Similarly, high-end nutritional shakes can cost over $3 per serving, equating to over $100 monthly for one daily nutrition shake. Preparing meals from scratch may not be feasible for those who work multiple jobs to make ends meet, as they may need more time or resources.

Some have suggested that semaglutide improves this situation and that promoting a "disease model" of obesity can allow overweight people to be treated as patients suffering from illness and not people who make poor life choices.

There is a severe problem at hand – obesity is just one aspect of the nutrition crisis that a growing number of people are facing. Inaccessibility to healthy foods and the abundance of unhealthy foods is not just a matter of gaining weight. It is a matter of shortened life expectancy due to various reasons such as nutrient deficiency, cardiovascular disease, hypertension, and diabetes.

These conditions can be caused by unhealthy processed foods, which can be prevented through a healthy diet. Merely reducing caloric intake is not sufficient to prevent any of these conditions. Instead, one needs to increase nutrient density while decreasing the density of unhealthy fats, sugar, and salt.

Is semaglutide merely masking the problem and making it less visually apparent? It is essential to consider whether we can truly solve the issue of obesity by simply prescribing weight loss drugs. Unfortunately, our patients often suffer from nutrient deficiencies due to their inability to afford healthy food, which can ultimately lead to shortened lifespans. This is primarily because they are overworked and underpaid.

The use of drugs for weight management might be a prolonged process, and it is essential for the public to understand that, just like any other ailment, you might have to continue taking it for the remainder of your life.

Our main objective should be to educate readers about the importance of nutrient-dense foods and provide recipes that make these foods more appealing to those who crave unhealthy foods due to stress.

While sharing recipes can make cooking and eating healthy foods more effortless, it is essential to note that it is only helpful if a person can afford the ingredients or has access to cooking facilities.

We must come together to address the rising public health concerns. One of the key steps towards this end is to improve the availability of fresh and healthy foods and accessible cooking facilities. While medication can help alleviate specific ailments, it cannot replace the importance of a balanced, nutritious diet.

Moreover, providing advice on healthy eating habits will only suffice if people can afford fresh foods. We need to take concrete steps towards making healthy food options more affordable and accessible for everyone and make cooking facilities readily available to ensure that people can prepare nutritious meals at home.

WE ARE NEVER TOO OLD TO LEARN NEW TRICKS

In January of 2024, KevinMD published my essay about an experience that reminded me of the importance of lifelong learning. I had a patient who was early in his gender transition—and I had to speak to him about a medical condition that may have been related to his uterus.

I was certainly not taught how to handle this when I attended medical school in the 1980s. This was partly due to an overall lack of education about bedside manners in my medical school. But there was also the problem that best practices for addressing transgender people were not widely known in mainstream culture at that time.

As we navigate the complexities of healthcare, it is essential to recognize the role of medical professionals in treating patients with respect and dignity. However, this is only sometimes the case. Many medical professionals lack adequate training to handle patients with empathy and compassion.

In this essay, I delve into the significance of providing medical professionals with better training to understand the importance of treating patients with respect and dignity. I also share my experiences where I had fallen short of treating patients with the respect they deserved, and the lessons I learned from those mistakes.

Every medical professional can learn from the experiences of others and become better equipped to handle patients with empathy and kindness.

Lessons From Treating a Transgender Patient

I was recently reminded that you always learn something from your patients, no matter how long your medical profession is. I was reminded of this when I had the opportunity to treat a young person in transition. I reviewed the chart before walking into the exam room. Among other things, it listed the patient's chief complaint (i.e., in this case, lower back pain), age of nineteen, female sex, and a female name for the patient.

As I entered the exam room, I assumed there had been a mistake with the chart. "I am sorry, I think I have the wrong chart," I said—maybe before I had even said hello. "You do not," the patient explained, with a tired expression as if they had made the same correction many times before.

It turns out that the patient was in the process of transitioning from female to male. He preferred to be called Marco. Marco had not legally changed his birth name yet, but he was—I later learned—engaged in separate medical care for gender dysmorphia. Surprisingly, my chart did not include any notes about Marco's transition. I was, therefore, caught unprepared.

I had treated transgender patients in the past, but this was the first time in 35 years of practicing medicine that I was treating a person in the early stages of transition (i.e., where their legal and major sexual characteristics had not yet caught up to the social transition to using a new name and pronouns).

I must admit that I fumbled for a minute but then collected myself and performed the required physical examination of the patient's back pain. Although I was missing the medical history regarding Marco's gender transition, I decided not to ask. I told myself it was not relevant to his back pain.

As human beings, we all have biases that are deeply ingrained in our psychology. They are the product of our life experiences and cultural and personal stereotypes with which we have grown up. Importantly, our biases may impact our thoughts, beliefs, and actions in ways we may not realize. By acknowledging our biases and consciously recognizing and questioning them, we can help prevent them from negatively affecting our decisions and behavior.

This increased self-awareness can lead to a more equitable and just society where people are judged based on their merits rather than their race, gender, religion, or other personal characteristics.

In Marco's case, I was driven by fear of not asking questions about his transition. My discomfort—born of my own biases—prevented me from providing the absolute best care at that moment because I failed to ask the questions that may have made me understand the patient's condition and build a better doctor/patient relationship.

After reviewing a preliminary lumbar X-ray and an MRI report, I recommended lumbar facet joint injections under fluoroscopic guidance. Physical therapy had been ineffective for Marco. We followed the surgical center's standard protocol to prepare the patient for the procedure. However, almost right away, my staff needed to learn how to proceed.

Several nurses approached me about obtaining the required pregnancy test. They did not know how to approach Marco about it. Sadly, I felt uneasy, too. I consulted the medical director to let them make a decision. The patient was then asked to provide a urine sample for a pregnancy test by one of our practitioners.

Marco wanted to be happier about the bureaucratic requirement. I am sure it felt unfair and unnecessary to him. My obvious discomfort in managing the patient did not help matters.

In truth, the experience left me questioning my competency and level of empathy. In the state of Florida, before renewing our medical licenses, the state requires medical doctors to take mandatory courses on sex trafficking, domestic violence, medical errors, and controlled substance prescriptions. Surprisingly, these courses still do not cover transgender issues, regardless of the medical specialty.

In hindsight, I realized I had so many questions I could not answer. What is the best way to document a patient's transgender status in a medical chart? How many questions about the specific treatment are appropriate? Medication histories are critical in a surgical setting, but what about other interventions? If a pregnancy test is required for a person identifying as male, what is the best way to explain that to the patient without disrespecting them?

Some doctors, I suspect, avoid specific topics and questions with transgender patients, particularly those who are in the early stages of transition. What might we be missing by failing to engage professionally and respectfully?

Doctors and other medical professionals would be in a better position to provide high-quality health care services if they possessed a comprehensive understanding of the medical implications that gender issues can have on the overall health of individuals.

By better grasping the various gender-related concerns that a patient may have, doctors can tailor their diagnosis, treatment, and care to meet each patient's specific needs, thereby enhancing the overall quality of care provided.

Medical training must evolve to better prepare doctors for this population in medical school and continuing education settings. This will ensure that doctors in the back half of their careers are as equipped with the appropriate protocols and pertinent medical information as the younger generations. The effective treatment of these patients demands it.

Is There a Class on How to Give Bad News?

One of my most educational experiences as an intern was the first time I saw a patient receive a terminal diagnosis. Unfortunately, it was something of a class in what not to do.

Too often, doctors are called upon to give patients devastating news. There is an argument to be made that these are our most important moments as doctors: the moment we must sit with a patient as they confront their mortality.

Yet, there is still no standardization or protocol for teaching this skill to medical students. How can we frame these pivotal moments in meaningful ways without offering false hope?

This essay first appeared in KevinMD in February of 2024.

A Intern's Journey in Delivering Tough Diagnoses

I was an intern who had recently graduated from medical school with little hands-on experience when the patient signaled me to his bedside. Initially, I did a double-take, wondering if the man would be asking for me. I glanced anxiously at the morning rounds as they hurried to the next patient. I'd just watched my attending physician present this patient's case, speaking about him as though he weren't there.

The attending didn't even look at the patient as he explained the severity of the patient's cancer, which I even realized was likely to be terminal. This was typical of our morning rounds: little to no communication with the patients displayed almost like museum exhibits.

Maybe the man recognized my look of concern and empathy for his condition in a sea of indifference. He could tell that I was uncomfortable with this presentation style. Perhaps he had somehow mistaken me for a more senior and experienced doctor. The patient insisted on seeing me for whatever reason, and I finally obliged.

"Give it to me straight," the man stated gravelly. "I somehow trust you. Tell me my prognosis."

I immediately went pale and broke out in a sweat. I nervously looked around. I was supposed to interact with patients a different way, according to the assignment rosters. Anything I said could interfere with his care team's plan.

"I-I am sorry," I stuttered. "You need to talk to the attending physician. I don't know the details."

However, looking at him, I paused. This man was not merely a demand to be fulfilled. He was a human being. Seeing the intensity and desperation of his eyes on me, I realized he did not just want information. He needed human connection.

I stayed with him for a few minutes, fussing around his bed and ensuring he was comfortable. It was all I could do. I didn't say much. Still, he felt better when I left. He looked more at peace.

A year later, while in my second year of residency, we received a fifty-year-old veteran experiencing atrophy in one of his hand muscles as the only complaint.

At first examination, the nerve conduction appeared normal. However, we found abnormal nerve transmission in his arms and leg muscles during his electromyogram, which is characteristic of motor neuron disease. Our attending told us sadly that he most likely had Amyotrophic Lateral Sclerosis (ALS). If he did, it would eventually kill him.

Our attending displayed sadness with us behind closed doors, but her demeanor with the patient was different. Perhaps no one had trained her to handle the complex emotions involved in giving someone a terminal diagnosis. She spoke brusquely, with a flat voice intonation, as she told the man that he probably had ALS and that if so, the prognosis was not good.

I watched the veteran's face change. For a moment, there was devastation. Then, it was replaced by anger. "You don't know what you're talking about!" the man roared, standing up indignantly. "I come in with a hand sprain, and you tell me I'm dying? You're all incompetent!" he shouted as he stormed out.

I watched the exchange in shock. The patient's reaction was unexpected, but the attending's impersonal mask as she spoke to the patient was just as uncomfortable to observe. What was the right way to deliver a grim diagnosis? I mused. Somewhat shocked, I realized I didn't know myself.

As a resident physician, I had never been given formal education on how to tell a patient they were dying. There were no lectures or classes on bedside manner. I had assumed that compassion and empathy would be, however, now I see that reality is more complicated.

The danger is that if the empathy level is high and there is no professional detachment, the interaction could become so overwhelming that doctors do not know how to handle their own feelings. Remaining cold and unfeeling in appearance could be considered a practical coping mechanism.

Patient denial of medical diagnoses is a complex problem for a physician. Anyone who has had a patient refuse to take their medication knows this. With the growing popularity of anti-vaccine movements that teach that sound, strong people don't get sick, this problem only appears to be getting worse.

A year after that veteran stormed out of our clinic, I saw him again. He was now confined to a wheelchair. He was dependent on an oxygen tank to breathe, and his speech was barely audible. It was a shocking transformation that left me profoundly moved and saddened.

I knew that there are few treatments for ALS, and so his denial probably hadn't played a role in his rapid decline. However, what if he had a condition that could be treated and had delayed or refused treatment because he didn't trust the diagnosis or the doctor?

I look back on the day of the veteran's diagnosis and wish he had received a more compassionate response. Had the attending appeared more concerned for their condition, would he have trusted her as that patient trusted me to tell him the truth all those years ago?

As a healthcare professional, I understand the importance of being upfront with my patients and helping them mentally prepare for a challenging diagnosis. I recognize the importance of guiding them to accept realistic expectations and protecting them from the dangers of having unfounded optimism that may lead them to attempt desperate measures or be preyed upon by unscrupulous people with useless alternative therapies.

Wanting to provide hope to suffering people is a natural human tendency. As doctors, however, this need is superseded by the responsibility to provide accurate and realistic information on the diagnosis, the prospects, and the recommended courses of action, so that patients can make informed decisions and come to terms with their challenges.

However, these critical directives do not preclude that the information be communicated with tact, compassion, understanding, and, most importantly, dignity.

When Doctors are Unprepared

A fter an earthquake shattered Haiti's capital city in 2010, I volunteered to join a team of doctors flying to my hospital to help with the recovery efforts. Upon arriving, however, I found that good intentions were not enough: most of us were woefully unprepared to practice disaster medicine in the field.

After KevinMD published this essay in February 2024, other doctors reached out to me and thanked me for validating their experiences. They had been in similar situations: volunteering to work in disaster zones, only to find themselves questioning how well their medical training had prepared them to work outside of the hospital setting.

In this essay, I argue that the extent to which modern medical training specializes doctors in being dependent on the infrastructure of modern hospitals and the ways in which we can augment our training to be prepared for a wider variety of situations need to be discussed.

From Pain Management to Port au Prince: A Doctor's Journey in Disaster Relief

As medical doctors, we think we can help alleviate physical suffering in almost any situation. When the 2010 earthquakes shattered Haiti's capital, I felt compelled to help. I had extensive pain management experience and training as a physiatrist. I thought I was ideally suited to lend a hand. At the time, this all seemed obvious. But I had never been in a disaster zone before, which made me hesitant.

Still, my heart pounding, I accepted a colleague's call for volunteers to go to Port au Prince on a humanitarian mission. I was exhilarated by the prospect of playing the hero. However, I soon learned that helping people in disaster circumstances is more complicated than I had anticipated. To begin with, I was shocked by the difficulties in just getting there. The group of doctors I traveled with and our medical supplies depended on donated private transportation to Haiti.

Moving large volumes of medical supplies is difficult most times. But when the transportation is inadequate and ten times smaller than what it should be, then things get interesting. We crammed our equipment first into a private jet belonging to a friend of one of the doctors. Then we transferred to another private jet lent to us by a random patron.

Upon arrival in Port au Prince, I soon realized how out-of-my-depth I was. I had been trained to practice medicine in a U.S. hospital setting. But here, no functional hospitals were left. Under these circumstances, I had yet to be trained to improvise or operate at a basic level. There were no options to abide by usual best practices. It dawned on me that I quickly needed to adapt so that I wouldn't accidentally do more damage to the patients I treated.

I found that the most critical patients were those with crush injuries, of which there were many. Untreated crush injuries have a high mortality. For this reason, one of the doctors on our team had come prepared to perform field amputations en masse. He had a bone saw and intravenous acetaminophen for pain but very little else. He seemed to know what he was doing. I certainly did not.

I felt relegated to what I felt competently that I could do: administer IV acetaminophen and monitor a patient to see if they were crashing. Therefore, I volunteered to help the surgeon, holding the fully conscious patients' hands, as my colleague amputated their dying limbs. Around us, diseases like cholera were rampant. I knew only how that would have been treated in the hospital. Fortunately, aid agencies had thought of this but needed help transporting clean water onto the island. They were struggling to stop people from drinking the contaminated water.

We gave oral rehydration solution and antibiotics to reduce mortality rates among the treated patients. However, I had to be taught to do this by field medics because it was not part of my training as a doctor. This experience was an impactful revelation of how woefully unprepared many doctors are to function outside of the particular range of circumstances in which they are taught to operate.

As doctors, we are taught to operate in the context of multidisciplinary teams. We are encouraged to specialize in knowledge, often learning little about how to treat conditions outside our range of expertise. We are taught to abide by best practices, but not when those become unavailable. We are rarely taught to improvise. Those in the medical profession should invest in intentional training in emergency field crises if they want to make a difference in helping in the world health crisis.

Otherwise, the time spent may be more about providing a warm but temporary sense of significance or, at worst, some posts on social media to broadcast their involvement. Medical degrees allow the treatment of almost any medical condition under most circumstances. But are we qualified to do so under extreme conditions? How many of us would be comfortable treating patients if our support systems broke down or if we were faced with impossibly limited supplies?

After my experience in Haiti, I also began to think about how equipped I was to handle the standard proverbial "Is there a doctor in the house?" emergencies. I don't know how to manage a heart attack on an airplane beyond administering CPR. I don't know how to care for a car accident victim beyond trying to stop bleeding and conducting a neurological assessment.

If we want to help in emergencies under sub-optimal circumstances, we must add field medicine to our repertoire. As the COVID-19 pandemic taught us, we cannot assume that best practices will always be available, even within our hospitals. While I was in Haiti, I found myself debilitated by overwhelming feelings of helplessness and despair. Witnessing the human tragedy around me made me question my abilities as a medical professional and face the limitations of my expertise.

In retrospect, this highlighted the need to have training in the psychological stresses of practicing medicine under these conditions. In the aftermath of our trip to Haiti, we received much credit for our volunteerism. I saw instances of some taking photographs of doctors helping patients, which were then splashed across hospital public relations pages. I know our efforts helped, but I wonder how much more impactful it could have been.

Nevertheless, genuine care and empathy when interacting with patients are transformative and have a healing effect under any circumstance. Trying to face the world's problems can be overwhelming, but we can cope when we strive to make a difference in our given sphere of influence. But we must be willing to adopt a willingness in humility to adapt and learn if we want to expand that area of influence. We should create and improve curricula at medical schools to practice in crisis locations. We should mentally prepare for the psychological stress we will face before traveling to emergencies outside our norm, but it must be done for the right reasons and with proper preparation.

THE HUMAN ELEMENT

The most powerful stories from my medical career are not about rare diseases or mystery diagnoses. They are the moments in which humanity is revealed in all of its sacred and unexpected complexity. I had some of my most potent experiences of revealing humanity in an electromyography lab.

At the time, electromyography was a procedure that required doctors to physically touch patients, often while alone in a room together. Under these circumstances, profound and unexpected truths about who my patients were as human beings were revealed.

In this essay, which was the impetus for assembling this book, I discuss what I believe to be the most crucial part of the art of medicine and my hopes and fears about how advancing technology may be used to revive or destroy the humanizing art of medicine.

Unlocking Compassion: Lessons from a Prison Clinic

The healing potential of human interaction should always be considered, particularly when practicing medicine. Early in my medical career, I worked in the electromyography laboratory at Charity Hospital, Louisiana State University. During my time there, I saw an astonishing variety of patients. Among other things, we were the hospital of choice for the nearby Louisiana State Penitentiary, Angola, or "The Alcatraz of the South." This prison was infamous for housing violent offenders.

I was still a somewhat inexperienced doctor the day I watched correctional officers bring this imposing man into my clinic. He was robust, muscular, and shackled from his neck down to his ankles. I watched, astonished, as it took the officers minutes to fully unbind him. Then, adding to my growing unease, they left me alone with him. By law, the correctional officers had to wait outside the room while I examined the prisoner. Unfortunately, it was my job to stick him with needles and administer other intrusive diagnostics to evaluate him. I noticed I was sweating as I set up the medical instruments. My hands were also shaking. However, surprisingly, I also noticed his hands were sweaty as well.

"Will this hurt, doc?" he asked in a profound yet fragile voice. "I do not like needles," he added.

I looked up into his face with a jerk, unable to disguise my surprise. In my mind's eye, I saw him looking back at me, growing angry and trying to make some desperate attempt to escape. Instead, I found him watching me with evident anxiety, the same as I might see in many other patients. His unease may have been augmented by very overt apprehension. But I found myself placing my trembling hand on his for comfort. "It will hurt," I said, "but not much," I reassured him.

The man took a deep breath, half a sigh of relief and half steeling himself. Unexpectedly, he shared, "I killed somebody," and "That's the reason I'm in Angola." My mouth went dry. I did not know how to respond. What could you say to that? I focused on the tests I was administering. Regardless of the unusual circumstances, I was finding it impossible to see this man as anything other than another patient. He was a nervous human being waiting for the needle. I wondered what circumstances he must have been in so that committing murder seemed necessary. His willingness to expose his fears increased my empathy for his situation.

As I spent more time in the lab during that period, I found that my work resulted in more of these atypical interactions and related introspections. Perhaps there was something about the fact that the work required physical touch. Also, the fact that many of the patients were unexpectedly afraid and felt better by sharing their feelings. They took this opportunity with me, a stranger, to show vulnerability and share their most profound burdens, perhaps because they considered a doctor to be a non-judgmental player.

As a healthcare professional, I have listened to countless stories from my patients. However, I must admit that at times, their stories leave me in disbelief, at times, in awe. It's incredible how much we can learn and appreciate about the people around us when they open up and share their experiences. Perspective is everything, and learning about someone's struggles and history provides a fantastic focus on appreciation. I often wonder, as I pass people on the street, about their stories and what roads they have traveled to be at the places they are at the moment.

The doctor-patient relationship is a unique bond built on trust, confidentiality, respect, and empathy. Patients often feel comfortable sharing their deepest concerns and fears with their health care providers, which can foster an atmosphere of honesty and openness in the relationship. Several factors contribute to this dynamic, including doctors' being trained to listen well and provide compassionate patient care. Additionally, patients may feel relieved knowing they can speak freely without fear of judgment or reprisal, perhaps for the first time in their lives.

This level of trust and vulnerability can be humbling and rewarding for health care providers, as they can provide support and guidance to those who need it most. Ultimately, the doctor-patient relationship is an essential aspect of health care, and it plays a crucial role in promoting healing and well-being for patients and their families.

In today's world, technology is advancing rapidly, and medicine is no exception. While technology has undoubtedly brought many benefits and improvements to the medical field, one must ask whether we are losing the art of medicine through a significant increase in the pace of medical care. The "art of medicine" is solidly based on the human connection between the patient and the doctor, considering the patient's unique circumstances and needs.

As technology and automated diagnostic capabilities become more prevalent in the medical field, it is essential to remember the importance of the human element in medicine. While technology can significantly impact diagnosis and treatment, the value of human interaction and empathy should be recognized. Doctors must remember that they treat a patient with a disease. By maintaining the art of medicine, we can ensure that patients receive the best care possible and that doctors can connect with their patients on a deeper level.

Conclusion

Becoming a physician was a decision I made with the knowledge that it was not an exact science but rather an art that required creativity, intuition, and a deep understanding of human nature. I was driven to develop my knowledge and skills and use them to benefit my patients and the wider community. This meant embracing the challenges and uncertainties inherent in the field of medicine and continually learning and adapting to new situations and technologies. Being a physician is not just a job but a calling that demands dedication, compassion, and a commitment to excellence.

The practice of medicine is a combination of both scientific knowledge and technical skills, as well as a deep understanding of human nature, empathy, and compassion. Healthcare providers must balance these elements to provide the best possible care to their patients.

In my over 30 years of practice, I have seen medicine evolve. I have also evolved myself as a human being. I have seen attitude shifts in society and in the medical community. Mostly, these changes have been for the better: we have learned more, and some of the patient-centered education and best practices I longed for in the 1990s are now a reality.

We must be mindful of how we proceed as doctors in the decades to come. We now have more opportunities for ongoing education, including learning how to engage with patients as human beings collaboratively to maximize well-being. We have more ways than ever before to reach and treat patients and more specialized knowledge of how to treat their minds and bodies.

Yet, we also face new and changing pressures. External pressures can make it difficult to be centered and fully present with patients in the exam room and to feel comfortable really taking the time to listen. It is up to us as individuals to fight the impulse to treat our patients as mere collections of laboratory values or items on an ever-growing to-do list.

The good news is that practicing medicine as a human art is its own reward. For me, at least, the interactions I have when I am fully present for my patients are what make the art of medicine worth practicing. These moments of connection far outweigh the stresses of modern practice.

I am sometimes disheartened to hear news that an increasing number of doctors are not encouraging their children to enter the medical field. While medicine was once considered the gold standard career for our children, many modern doctors consider the field too stressful and insufficiently rewarding. Could this be because the growth of external pressures squeezes out the time and space we feel we have for the human connection?

Efficient communication and attentive listening are essential in medicine, not just diagnosing and treating ailments. The art of medicine necessitates physicians to treat the complete individual, not solely the disease or condition they may be suffering from.

The art of medicine is about building a relationship between the physician and the patient, one that is based on trust, respect, and understanding. It involves providing care tailored to each patient's needs, considering their unique circumstances and preferences.

In summary, the art of medicine is a holistic healthcare approach involving technical skills, empathy, compassion, and effective communication. It requires physicians to treat patients as whole persons and build meaningful relationships with them.

As we move into the future, let us work together to ensure that technology

is used to restore the human art of medicine—not to undermine it. Let us ensure that AI is used under the supervision of doctors who make collaborative treatment decisions, considering their patients' desires and emotions. Let us ensure that faster diagnoses mean more time spent speaking with patients, not less.

If we can move forward together conscientiously, we can create a brighter future for patients and doctors everywhere.

About the Author

Dr. Francisco Torres is the author of seven books, including Epigenetics and the Psychology of Weight Loss, Keep Kicking Frisco, Keep Kicking, and Dr. T's Drop the Fat Cookbook. He writes regularly for KevinMD and DoximityOpMed. He is a physiatrist in Clearwater, FL. He is affiliated with multiple hospitals in the area, including Largo Medical Center, Mease Countryside Hospital, Morton Plant Hospital, Tampa Community Hospital, and Morton Plant North Bay Hospital.

Dr. Torres received his medical degree from the University of Puerto Rico School of Medicine and has practiced for 31 years. He speaks multiple languages, including Spanish. He specializes in pain and sports medicine (non-surgical) and is experienced in physical medicine and rehabilitation, pain management, electrodiagnostic testing, musculoskeletal disorders, and age management.

When he's not treating patients or writing, Dr. Torres enjoys playing the violin and taking long walks on the beach with his dog, Gaudete. He hopes his books will help patients in the same way he has been helped by his numerous teachers and life experiences across the decades.

Keep Kicking Frisco, Keep Kicking: Letting Go of Fear, Anxiety, and Panic

Francisco Torres was an anxious child. It's easy to understand why when you read about his family's history with the Spanish Civil War, Draconian religious schools, and mental illness. After surviving multiple brushes with death early in life, Dr. Torres set out to conquer his anxiety. "Keep Kicking, Frisco" is equal parts memoir, history, adventure, and comedy. Dr. Torres gives an insider view on conquering panic disorder through a combination of therapy, self-help, and placing himself in situations where panic could have proven fatal.

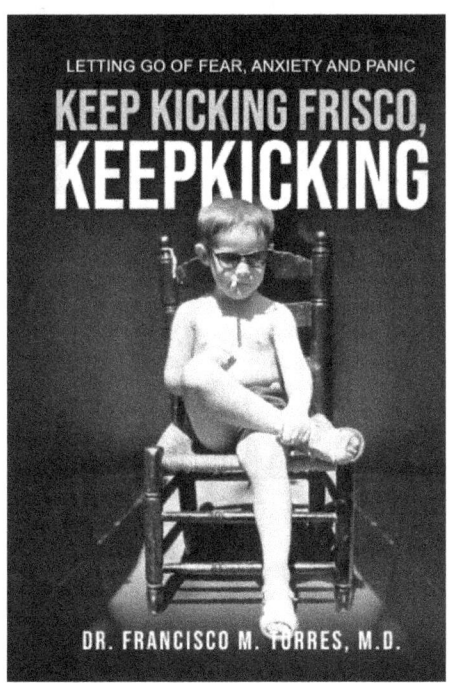

Provocative Thoughts for Daily Living

Dr. Francisco Torres believes that philosophy has a key place in the practice of medicine and in determining its role in society. In a series of powerful vignettes, Dr. Torres sparks reflection and reevaluation. In "Provocative Thoughts for Daily Living," he leverages both his personal and professional experiences in healthcare to explore the deeper questions that arose amid his own journey to self-discovery. His meditations, collected here, are designed to provoke transformative and inspirational ideas in the reader.

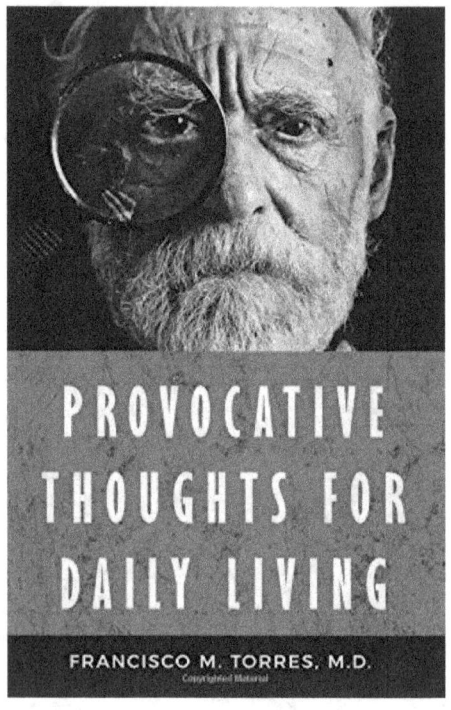

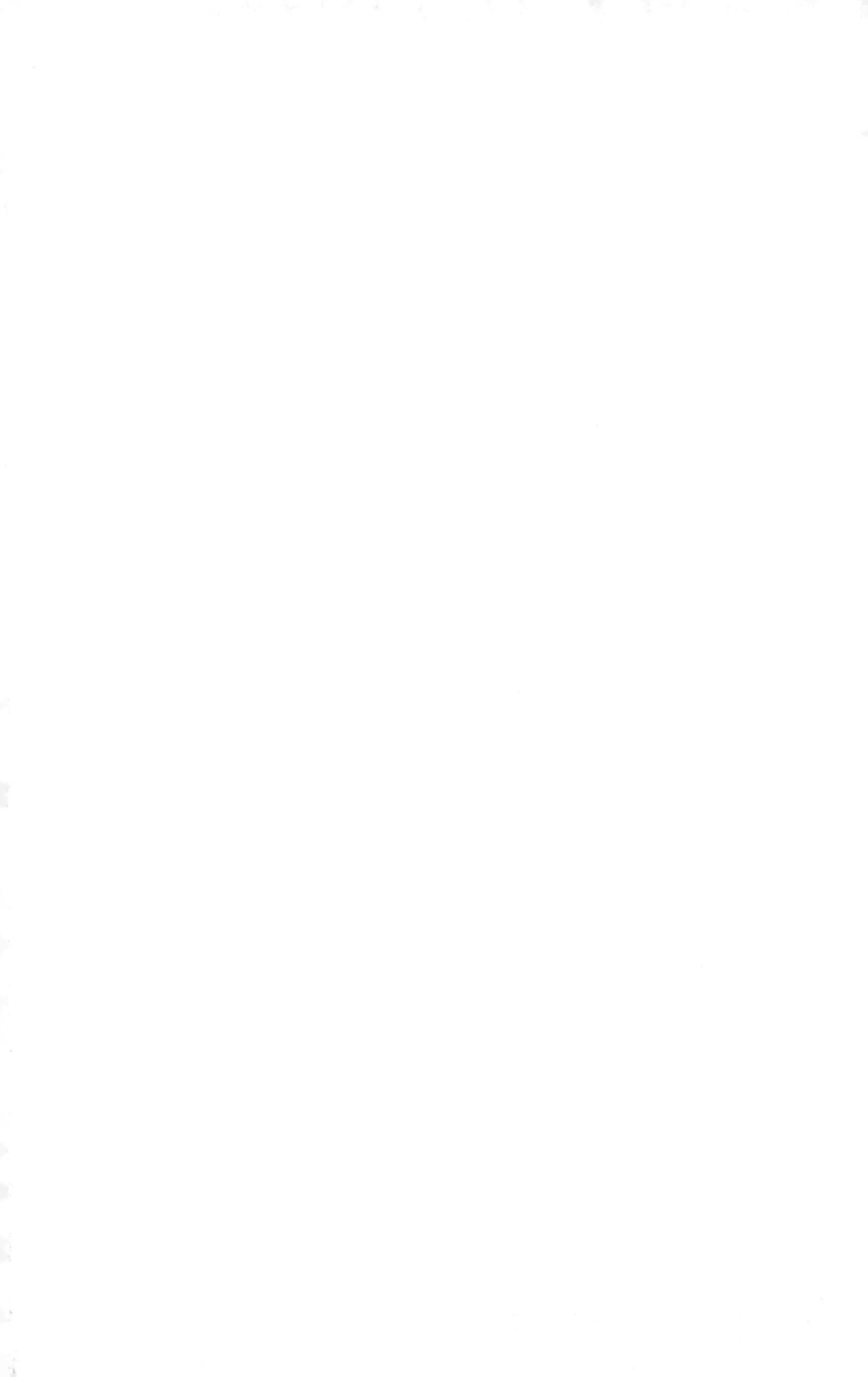

www.ingramcontent.com/pod-product-compliance
Lightning Source LLC
Chambersburg PA
CBHW050334010526
44119CB00004B/148